Syntropy and Homeopathy

Ulisse Di Corpo

www.sintropia.it

Copyright © 2018 Ulisse Di Corpo

ISBN: 9781730835292

INDEX

Introduction	1
The flap of a butterfly's wing	15
Retrocausality	53
Intuitions	67
Epilogue	75

INTRODUCTION

In the forties, many researchers and scientists came to the discovery of syntropy. The mathematician Luigi Fantappiè coined the term *Syntropy*, the psychiatrist Wilhelm Reich named it *Orgone*, the evolutionary palaeontologist Teilhard de Chardin called it the *Omega Point*. Wilhelm Reich was arrested and died in prison for a heart attack a few days before being released. His laboratories were destroyed and all his books burned, probably the worst case of censorship in the history of the United States. Teilhard de Chardin was exiled to China, he also died of a heart attack. Immediately after the Vatican issued a decree that forbade all his works and imposed their withdrawal from libraries and bookstores because: *"they offend the Catholic doctrine"* and to *"defend the spirits, especially of the young people, from the dangers of the works of Father Teilhard de Chardin and his disciples."* Also Luigi Fantappiè died of a heart attack, in that same period, in July 1956. His *Theory of the Physical and Biological World* was withdrawn from all the libraries and became unavailable. All the documents and works relating to syntropy were removed from his private archive.

Homeopathy is also the subject of similar attacks. In Italy the famous TV science journalist Piero Angela (i.e. he has no university degree or scientific background) reiterates that *"homeopathy is fresh water"*, *"pseudoscience"* or even *"magic practice"* and continually underlines that it does not have any scientific validity. *"It's a placebo effect, this is what the scientific community says."* Angela points out that: *"For Rita Levi Montalcini* (an Italian Nobel laureate) *homeopathy is a potentially harmful non-cure because it takes away patients from other valid treatments"* and that *"for Renato Dulbecco* (another Italian Nobel laureate) *it is a matter of no value."* Lately the attacks on homeopathy have intensified; the main accusations are that homeopathy has no scientific basis and the effects reported by its users are exclusively due to the placebo effect.

In an initiative against the hoaxes of the Federation of the Medical Order, the FNOMCeO, writes[1] that *"at present there is no scientific evidence or biological plausibility that prove the validity of the mechanisms of functioning of homeopathy such as the 'Simillimum' according to which the homeopathic remedy that when given to a healthy person produces the symptom of the disease in question cures the disease. There is no scientific evidence of the principle of 'dilution', known by practitioners as 'dynamisation' or 'potentisation', which is a process in which a substance is diluted and then vigorously shaken in a process called 'succession'. In fact, several studies conducted with a rigorous methodology have shown that no pathology gets improvements or healings thanks to homeopathic remedies. At best, the effects are similar to those obtained with a placebo (an inert substance). On the other hand there are numerous personal testimonies that refer to therapeutic successes due to homeopathy, but these can easily be explained with the placebo effect, with the normal course of the disease or with the expectation of the patient. The placebo effect has a well-known neurophysiological basis and also works on animals and children, but its use in therapy is ethically questionable and debated. On the other hand, the supposed mechanisms of functioning of homeopathy are contrary to the laws of physics and chemistry."*

The goal of this book is to demonstrate how the functioning mechanisms of homeopathy are perfectly compatible with the laws of physics.

For years there have been ferocious attacks on those who study the laws of physics that are compatible with homeopathy: censorship at conferences, the impossibility of publishing, loss of academic positions and funding.

In our professional life we have had the opportunity to experience this censorship. Our Syntropy page has been censored by Wikipedia,

---

[1] dottoremaeveroche.it/lomeopatia-ha-effetti-scientificamente-dimostrati

it has been removed and cannot be re-inserted. Now it points to a completely different concept: Negentropy. When Antonella Vannini developed the experimental procedures that test the theory of syntropy, she became the target of personal attacks, professors in the academia asked for her expulsion from the university and none of her tutors were present at the discussion of her PhD dissertation before the national commission. They were all terrified at the idea of being associated with such a forbidden theory. Several times I have been approached by people who have told me to stop working on syntropy. One of these came with a letter from Feynman in response to one of Fantappiè, and ordered me to stop working on syntropy because I had become a *"persona non grata."*

A scientific note is at this point necessary.

The energy-mass equation ($E = mc^2$), which we all associate with Einstein's 1905 theory of special relativity, was published by Oliver Heaviside in 1890[2], by Henri Poincaré in 1900[3] and by Olinto De Pretto in 1904[4]. Olinto De Pretto presented it to the Veneto Institute of Sciences in an essay with a preface by the astronomer and senator Giovanni Schiaparelli. It seems that the equation arrived to Einstein through his father Hermann who was responsible for the lighting systems in Verona and that, as director of the *"Privileged Electrical Enterprise Einstein"*, he had frequent contacts with the Fonderia De Pretto that produced the turbines for the production of electricity.

However, the energy-mass equation has a problem: it cannot be generalized because it does not take into account speed, which is also a form of energy. In 1905 Einstein solved this limit by adding, in the

---

[2] Auffray J.P., *Dual origin of E=mc2*: http://arxiv.org/pdf/physics/0608289.pdf
[3] Poincaré H,. *Arch. néerland. sci.* 2, 5, 252-278 (1900).
[4] De Pretto O., *Lettere ed Arti*, LXIII, II, 439-500 (1904), Reale Istituto Veneto di Scienze.

equation, the momentum and thus obtaining the energy-momentum-mass equation:

$$E^2 = m^2c^4 + p^2c^2$$

In this equation energy is squared (E^2) and in the momentum (p) we have time. A square root must therefore be used and consequently there are always two solutions: positive-time energy and negative-time energy.

Negative time energy implies the existence of retrocausality: the future that affects the past. This was considered impossible! To solve this paradox, Einstein suggested to remove the momentum, since the speed of physical bodies is practically nil compared to the speed of light. Considering the momentum equal to zero ($p = 0$), we return to the $E=mc^2$.

However, in 1924 the spin of the electrons was discovered, an angular momentum, a rotation of the electron on itself at a speed close to that of light. In atomic physics the momentum cannot be considered equal to zero and consequently the extended energy-momentum-mass equation of special relativity is required. The first equation that combined special relativity and quantum mechanics is dated 1926, by the physicists Oskar Klein and Walter Gordon. This equation has two solutions: a retrocausal (advanced waves) and a causal (delayed waves). The second equation, formulated in 1928 by Paul Dirac, has two solutions: electrons and neg-electrons (now positrons) that propagate backwards-in-time. The existence of positrons was experimentally demonstrated in 1932 by Carl Andersen.

However, Heisenberg and Bohr, both strongly charismatic physicists and with a prominent position in the institutions and academic world, imposed that only causality could be taken into consideration. From that moment, anyone who ventured into the study of retrocausality was discredited, lost the academic position, funding, the ability to publish and intervene at conferences.

In 1941 Luigi Fantappiè found himself struggling with the dual energy solution. Fantappiè was a mathematician and he could not accept that physicists had arbitrarily rejected half of the solutions of the fundamental equations. Listing the properties of the causal and retrocausal solution Fantappiè discovered that the causal solution is governed by the law of *entropy* (from the Greek words: *en*=diverging and *tropos*=tendency), while the retrocausal solution is governed by a symmetrical law that Fantappiè named *syntropy* (combining the Greek words: *syn*=converging and *tropos*=tendency). Causality involves diverging energy and the tendency towards dissipation and cooling of bodies, and it is identified with the famous second law of thermodynamics, also known as the law of thermal death or entropy. On the contrary, retrocausality implies converging energy, increasing temperatures, differentiation, complexity and the formation of structures and organizations. Listing these properties, Fantappiè discovered the mysterious qualities of life and in 1942 he published a booklet entitled *"The Unitary Theory of the Physical and Biological World"* in which he suggested that the physical-material world is governed by the law of entropy and causality, while the biological world is governed by the law of syntropy and retrocausality and that life must always tend to lower entropy and to increase syntropy.

But negative time energy is invisible, since we cannot see the future! The energy-momentum-mass equation posits the existence of a visible reality (causal and entropic) and an invisible reality (retrocausal and syntropic).

An example in physics is provided by gravity. We continually experience gravity, but we cannot see it. According to the energy-momentum-mass equation, gravity is a force that diverges backwards-in-time, therefore for us, moving forward in time, it is a converging force and it is invisible because it propagates from the future. The fact that gravity is invisible is known to all, but that it propagates from the future is known to few people.

How can we test this hypothesis? It is quite simple: if it propagates from the future its speed must be higher than that of light.

Tom van Flandern (1940-2009), an American astronomer specialized in celestial mechanics, has developed a series of procedures in order to test this hypothesis, measuring the velocity of propagation of gravity[5,6,7].

In the case of light, which has a limited speed of 300,000 kilometres per second, we observe the phenomenon of aberration. For example, the sunlight takes about 500 seconds to reach the Earth. Thus, when it arrives on the Earth, we see the Sun in the position of the sky that it occupied 500 seconds before. This difference amounts to about 20 seconds of arc, a large amount for astronomers. The light of the Sun hits the Earth from a slightly displaced angle and this displacement is called aberration.

If the speed of propagation of gravity is finite, one would expect to observe aberration in gravity measurements. Gravity should be maximal in the position that the Sun occupied when gravity left the Sun. But observations indicate that there is no detectable delay in the propagation of gravity from the Sun to the Earth. The direction of the gravitational pull of the Sun is exactly towards the position in which the Sun is located, not towards a previous position, and this shows that the speed of propagation of gravity is infinite.

Van Flandern also notes that gravity has some particular properties. One of these is that its effect on a body is independent of its mass and that the bodies fall into a gravitational field with the same acceleration, regardless of whether they are heavy or light.

---

[5] Van Flander T. (1996), *Possible New Properties of Gravity*, Astrophysics and Space Science 244:249-261.
[6] Van Flander T. (1998), *The Speed of Gravity What the Experiments Say*, Physics Letters A 250:1-11.
[7] Van Flandern T. and Vigier J.P. (1999), *The Speed of Gravity – Repeal of the Speed Limit*, Foundations of Physics 32:1031-1068.

Another property is the infinite extent of the gravitational force. The extension cannot be infinite when the forces propagate forward-in-time, at a finite speed. The other curious property of gravity is its instantaneous propagation, which can only be explained if we accept that gravity is a force that diverges backwards-in-time.

The fundamental equations lead to describe life as a system in-between the visible and the invisible, entropy and syntropy.

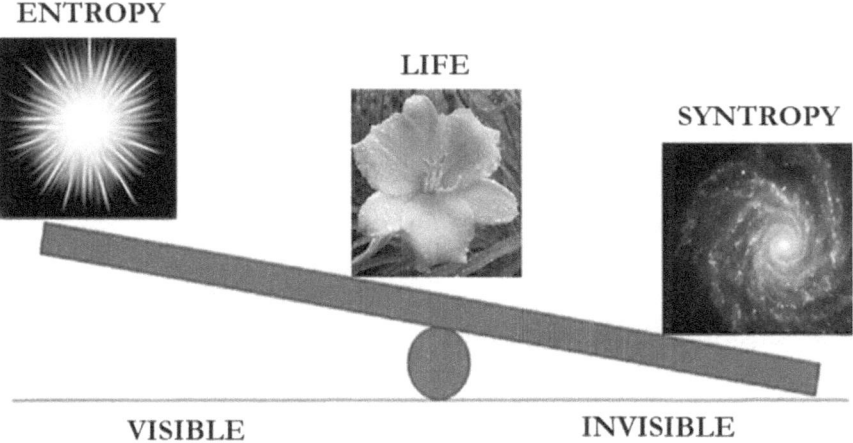

The first law of thermodynamics states that energy is a unity that cannot be created or destroyed, but only transformed, and the energy-momentum-mass equation shows that this unity is made of two components: a visible and an invisible one, one entropic and one syntropic, one causal and the other retrocausal. For this reason we can write that the unity of energy is equal to the sum of entropy and syntropy:

$$1 = Entropy + Syntropy$$

and in the same way that syntropy is the complement of entropy:

$$Syntropy = 1 - Entropy$$

This is deeply different from negentropy which is instead defined as the opposite of entropy (the negative of entropy):

$$negentropy = - entropy$$

However, Fantappiè failed to provide experimental evidence of his theory. In fact, the experimental method requires the manipulation of causes before observing their effects. This limits the scientific and experimental investigation to causality and prevents the study of all that is retrocausal and syntropic.

Lately Random Event Generators (REG) have become available. REG systems allow to perform experiments in which causes are manipulated in the future and the effects are studied in the present.

The first experimental study in this direction dates back to 1997, it was performed by Dean Radin of the ION (Institute of Noetic Sciences)[8]. Radin measured heart rate, skin conductance, and blood pressure in subjects who were shown a blank screens for 5 seconds followed by images that, based on a random event generator, could be calm or emotional. Radin observed a significant arousal (activation) of the parameters of the autonomic nervous system, before the presentation of emotional images. In 2003, Spottiswoode and May, of the Cognitive Science Laboratory, replicated these experiments carrying out a series of controls in order to study possible artifacts and alternative explanations. The results confirmed those already obtained by Radin, of the activation of the parameters of the autonomic nervous system before the presentation of emotional stimuli[9]. Similar results have been obtained by other

---

[8] Radin D.I. (1997), *Unconscious perception of future emotions: An experiment in presentiment*, Journal of Scientific Exploration, 11(2): 163-180.
[9] Spottiswoode P (2003) e May E, *Skin Conductance Prestimulus Response: Analyses, Artifacts and a Pilot Study*, Journal of Scientific Exploration, 2003, 17(4): 617-641.

authors, always using the parameters of the autonomic nervous system, for example: McCratly, Atkinson and Bradely[10], Radin and Schlitz[11] and May, Paulinyi and Vassy[12].

Daryl Bem, a psychologist and professor at the Cornell University, describes nine classical experiments in psychological literature, however, conducted in a time-reverse mode so as to obtain the effects before rather than after the stimulus.[13] For example, in a classic priming experiment, the subject is asked to judge whether the image is positive (pleasant) or negative (unpleasant) by pressing a button as quickly as possible. The reaction time (TR) is recorded. Just before the positive or negative image a word is presented briefly, below the threshold (i.e. in a way not perceptibly at the conscious level). This word is called *"prime"* and it has been observed that subjects tend to respond more quickly when the former is congruent with the image that follows (whether it is a positive image or a negative image), while reactions become longer when they are not congruent (for example, the word is positive while the image is negative). In the *retro-priming* experiments, the usual stimulus procedure occurs later, rather than before the subject responds, based on the hypothesis that this "inverse" procedure can influence retrocausally the responses. Experiments were conducted on more than 1,000 subjects, and they showed retrocausal effects with statistical significance of $p=1,34/10^{11}$ (one possibility among

---

[10] McCratly R (2004), Atkinson M e Bradely RT, *Electrophysiological Evidence of Intuition: Part 1*, Journal of Alternative and Complementary Medicine; 2004, 10(1): 133-143.
[11] Radin DI (2005) e Schlitz MJ, *Gut feelings, intuition, and emotions: An exploratory study*, Journal of Alternative and Complementary Medicine, 2005, 11(4): 85-91.
[12] May EC (2005), Paulinyi T e Vassy Z, *Anomalous Anticipatory Skin Conductance Response to Acoustic Stimuli: Experimental Results and Speculation about a Mechanism*, The Journal of Alternative and Complementary Medicine. August 2005, 11(4): 695-702.
[13] Bem D (2011), *Feeling the future: Experimental evidence for anomalous retroactive influences on cognition and affect*, Journal of Personality and Social Psychology, Jan 31, 2011.

134,000,000,000 to be mistaken when affirming the existence of the retrocausal effect).

The syntropy theory explains these results in the following way: *"Since life is nourished by syntropy, the parameters of the autonomic nervous system that supports vital functions must react in advance to future stimuli."*

As part of her PhD thesis in cognitive psychology, Antonella Vannini conducted four experiments using heart rate measurements in order to study the retrocausal effect.

Each experimental trial was divided into 3 phases:

Phase 1 Presentation of stimuli and measurement of heart rate				Phase 2 Choice	Phase 3 Random selection
Blue	Green	Red	Yellow	Blue/Green/Red/Yellow	Red
					Target
4 seconds HR01 HR02 HR03 HR04	4 seconds HR01 HR02 HR03 HR04	4 seconds HR01 HR02 HR03 HR04	4 seconds HR01 HR02 HR03 HR04		Feedback

Phase 1, presentation, in which 4 colours are shown one after the other on the computer screen. Each colour is shown for exactly 4 seconds. The subject is invited to look at the colours, and during the presentation the heart rate is measured. For each colour 4 heart rate measurements are recorded: one every second.

Phase 2, choice, in which an image with 4 coloured bars is shown in order to allow the subject (using the mouse) to indicate the colour that he thinks the computer will select in the third phase.

Phase 3, target, in which the computer randomly selects the colour (target) and shows it in full screen.

The hypothesis was as follows: in the presence of the retrocausal effect, a difference should be observed between heart rates measured in phase 1 in correlation with the target colour selected in phase 3. The presentation of the target colour (phase 3) is considered the cause of the differences observed in phase 1.

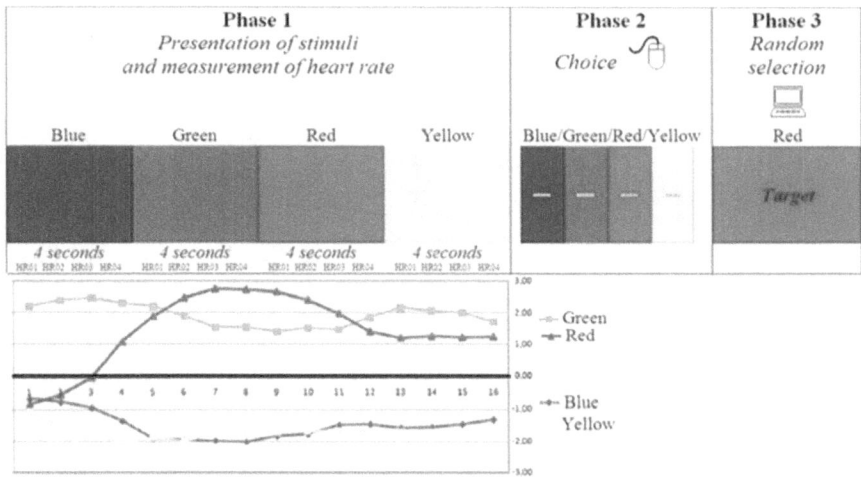

Effect seen in one subject

In the absence of the retrocausal effect, the heart rate lines associated with each colour of the target stimulus must vary around the 0.00 line. Instead, a marked difference is observed. Some subjects show an increase in heart rate when the target colour is blue and a reduction in heart rate when the target is green. Others show a pattern that is exactly the opposite. Performing the data analysis within each subject the retrocausal effect emerges with strong values of statistical significance. On the other hand, when the analysis is conducted in a classical way, adding together the effects observed among several subjects, opposite effects subtract and cancel each other out. This has shown that when studying retrocausal effects, parametric statistic techniques such as the Analysis of Variance (ANOVA) or Student's t do not show the effect, whereas non-parametric techniques such as Chi Squared and Fisher's exact test are able to see the effect. This is consistent with the division that Stuart Mill made in 1843, in his book *A System of Logic*, between the methodology of differences and the methodology of concomitant variations. Mill showed that causality can be studied using:

The <u>methodology of differences</u>: "*If in two groups initially similar an element of difference is introduced, the differences that can be observed can be attributed only to this single element that has been introduced.*"
The <u>methodology of concomitant variations</u>: "*When two phenomena vary concomitantly, one phenomenon may be the cause of the other or they are both united by the same cause.*"

The study of syntropic phenomena requires the use of the method of concomitant variations. This method does not imply the calculation of differences (i.e. means and variances), but only of frequencies and can therefore be used even when quantitative data are not available. It also allows to analyse an unlimited number of variables together. The method of concomitant variations is suitable for working on complexity, combining quantitative and qualitative, objective and subjective.[14]

But how does syntropy explain the mechanism of action of homeopathy?

The energy-momentum-mass equation shows that syntropy is available in the quantum level of matter. A question then arises spontaneously: how does syntropy move from the quantum level of matter to the macroscopic level of our physical reality, transforming inorganic matter into organic matter? In 1925 the physicist Wolfgang Pauli (1900-1958) discovered the hydrogen bridge (or hydrogen bond) in the water molecule. The hydrogen atoms of the water molecule are in an intermediate position between the sub-atomic (quantum) and molecular (macrocosm) levels, and provide a bridge that allows syntropy (cohesive forces) to flow from the micro to the

---

[14] See: www.amazon.com/dp/1520326637 e www.sintropia.it/sintropia.ds.zip

macro. The hydrogen bond increases the cohesive forces (syntropy) and makes water different from all other liquids, with cohesive forces ten times more powerful than the van der Waals forces that hold the other liquids together. Because of these remarkable cohesive forces, water exhibits abnormal properties. For example, when it freezes it expands, it becomes less dense and floats; on the contrary, the other liquids when they freeze contract, become denser and heavier and sink. The singularity of water lies in its attractive and cohesive properties (typical of the law of syntropy). The other molecules that make up hydrogen bonds (for example, ammonia) do not reach such high cohesive properties and therefore cannot build large-scale networks and structures, as it is the case with water. The hydrogen bond allows syntropy to flow from the subatomic level to the level of the macrocosm and makes water essential for life. Ultimately, water is the life-giving lymph, which provides syntropy. If life should ever start on another planet, surely water would be needed. According to syntropy water is an essential element for the manifestation and evolution of any biological structure.

It should be noted that hydrogen bonds also work in the opposite direction. Beside allowing syntropy to flow from the micro to the macro, they allow information to flow from the macro to the micro, informing syntropy, the attractor.

When working with causality, a bigger cause must be used to achieve a bigger effect. This is due to the fact that causality diverges and tends to dissipate. On the contrary, when working with retrocausality, the effect is amplified by the attractor. The smaller is the cause (the active ingredient), the more it can be amplified and the greater is the effect.

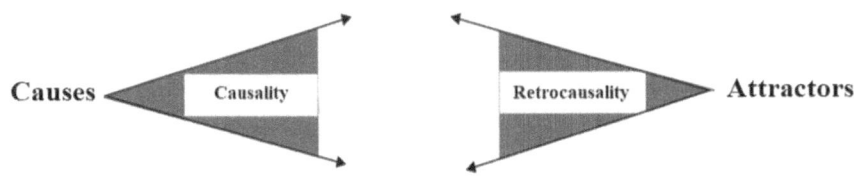

This strangeness of the attractors was first enunciated in 1963 by the meteorologist Edward Lorenz, who discovered that when it comes to water (which is the case in meteorology) a small variation can produce an effect that amplifies. To describe this situation Lorenz coined the famous phrase: " *The flap of a butterfly's wing in the Amazon can cause a hurricane in the United States.*" For this to happen it is necessary that the small flap (the active principle) is in line with the attractor. Otherwise entropy prevails and the small energy of the flap disperses into nothingness. An active principle which is in line with the attractor is amplified, on the contrary an active principle which is not in line with the attractor becomes nil.

The hydrogen bond operates in both directions: from the micro to the macro, amplifying the effect, and from the macro to the micro informing the attractor. The moment we insert into water the similar, the simillimum, of what we want to cure, its information (thanks to the dynamisation) goes into the quantum level and informs the attractor (syntropy). The greater the dilution, the greater will be the contribution of the attractor and the amplification of the effect.

1

THE FLAP OF A BUTTERFLY'S WING

In an interview titled *"The flap of a butterly's wing in the Amazon can cause a hurricane in the United States"* published in the journal *"Il Medico Omeopata"* (The Homeopathic Doctor) of July 2013 (year XVII number 53) Ulisse Di Corpo (UDC) was interviewed by Dr. Maurizio Paolella (*Q*), a unicist homeopathic doctor. The following text is an updated and revised version of this interview which focused on how syntropy can explain the mechanism of action of homeopathic remedies.

Q: I'd like to first know something about your studies and how you arrived to Fantappiè.

UDC: I discovered Fantappiè in a non-linear way. When I was eighteen, I had an intuition. I had always been an atheist; but this approach did not allow me to understand the strong and emotionally intense feelings which I was undergoing. At the age of sixteen, I participated to an exchange study experience of one year in the United States. I lived in Jefferson City Missouri with American families. Unlike my expectations, I experienced a strong existential crisis, accompanied by feelings of depression. This crisis went on for a couple of years, since April 1977 when my intuition lead me to what I now call *"The Theory of Vital Needs."* I saw the need for a new level of reality, I suddenly realized that we are not made only of matter and energy, but that there is a third level, which at the time I named the *feeling of life*, with properties symmetrical to those of physical energy. Instead of diverging it converges. Instead of propagating forward-in-time it had to propagate backward-in-time. This insight was crucial, since it lead me to the formulation of the *"Vital Needs Theory"* which enabled me to solve my existential crisis and my feelings of depression. Although I was particularly gifted in math, I chose to work on this intuition enrolling in the faculty of psychology, rather than that of engineering, physics or mathematics, which would have been my natural fields. The only professor who agreed to follow me in my thesis was an astrophysicist, Eliano Pessa. In my thesis I developed the Vital Needs Theory and the properties of this additional level. Briefly the Vital Needs Theory, in addition to material needs, posits the existence of needs for meaning and love. When a need is dissatisfied an alarm bell is triggered, such as hunger and thirst for the material needs and anguish for the dissatisfaction of the need for love, and depression for the dissatisfaction of the need for meaning. In this thesis it became clear that the third level which I added was a kind of negative-time energy. Alongside the traditional energy that we all know, for example, light that radiates from a light bulb, I speculated that a symmetrical energy which propagates from the future was providing us with the feeling of life. This energy, for us convergent, radiates from attractors which are in the future. This additional level allowed me to explain the feeling of life and consciousness, depression and anxiety and to solve the existential crisis that gripped me at that time.

Despite my enthusiasm for the Vital Needs Theory, reactions were of total disinterest. I finished the faculty of psychology disappointed and decided to enrol in a PhD in statistics and social research. I showed my thesis to the Dean of the Faculty of statistics, Vittorio Castellano, who told me that I had been working on the theory of "syntropy" of the mathematician Luigi Fantappiè. He offered to become my tutor for the final dissertation.

Luigi Fantappiè's publications on syntropy were impossible to find, they were not present in the libraries or book stores. I therefore went on by myself, without knowing what Fantappiè had written. Finally, in 1992 a small editor reprinted *"The Unitary Theory of the physical and biological world"* that Fantappiè had published in 1942. This work starts from the fundamental equations that combine quantum mechanics with special relativity. Since these equations are quadratic the solutions are always two: one with positive time and one with negative time. Physicists had rejected the negative time solution, since it makes no sense to have causes acting from the future, and since it contradicts the law of causality according to which causes must always precede their effects.

The positive time solution, was instead accepted since it describes classical causality, that acts forward-in-time, where causes always precede their effects.

Luigi Fantappiè (1901-1956) was considered one of the foremost mathematicians of the 20th century. He graduated at the age of 21 from the most exclusive Italian university, "La Normale Di Pisa", with a dissertation on pure mathematics, and became a full professor at the age of 27. During his university years he was a roommate of Enrico Fermi, worked with Werner Heisenberg, exchanged correspondence with Richard Feynman, and in April 1950 he was invited by Robert Oppenheimer to become a member of the exclusive Institute for Advanced Study in Princeton and work with Albert Einstein and other notable scholars. As a mathematician Fantappiè could not accept that physicists had taken the liberty to reject half of the solutions of the fundamental equations of the universe. Therefore, he began to work on the mathematical properties of these solutions and found that those which describe energy that diverges forward-in-time are governed by the law of entropy, where energy tends to diverge toward homogeneity. On the contrary, the backward-in-time solution, which for us is energy that converges and attracts, leads to increase differentiation, complexity, order and to the creation of structures.

Listing the mathematical properties of the backward-in-time energy solution, Fantappiè realized that they coincide with the properties of living systems. In his *Unitary Theory of the Physical and Biological World* Fantappiè suggests that the physical-chemical world follow the entropic positive time energy solution, whereas the biological world follows the negative time energy solution, where causality acts backward-in-time and it is governed by a law symmetrical to entropy that Fantappiè named syntropy, from the Greek *syn*=converging and *tropos*=tendency. Life, in essence, says Fantappiè, instead of being caused by the past is attracted by the future!

Q: A few more words on Fantappiè

UDC: Fantappiè was considered one of the great geniuses of the last century. He applied mathematics mainly to physics and he believed that mathematics contained a principle of reality. He could not accept the widespread habit among physicists, to use only those parts of the equations that were convenient. Equations had to be considered in their entirety. Fantappiè reminded that if the great book of nature is written in mathematical characters, as it was believed by Galileo, one must consider all the solutions.

The negative time solution was inconvenient since it introduces in physics the concept of final causality which contradicts the idea that causes must always precede their effects. According to the fundamental equations, causality is symmetrical there is as much forward causality as backward-in-time causality. Not only the biological world, but all of the universe would result from the continuous interaction of causality and retrocausality.

But the idea of retrocausality, which acts from the future was brutally censored. Fantappiè's books and papers on syntropy were censored, his theory on syntropy was degraded to a philosophy of an eccentric mathematician. He was accused of not having produced experimental evidences of his theory. The experimental method requires that causes be in the past. So, on the one hand the idea of retrocausality was rejected and on the other hand no experimental evidence could be provided. Fantappiè's theory fell soon into oblivion.

Furthermore, in physics the positive time and negative time solutions predict the same results, and it is therefore impossible to distinguish whether the effects which are observed depend from classical causality or retrocausality. For example, antimatter should flow backward-in-time, but it is impossible to establish whether antimatter actually flows forward or backward-in-time.

The situation is different in biology. In living systems anticipatory reactions are continuously observed, exactly as predicted by the theory of syntropy. The theory of syntropy assumes that life is nourished by syntropy and therefore the parameters of the vital processes must manifest reactions before their causes. These strange anticipatory reactions have been observed in all the living systems: individuals, cells, and also with organic molecules. The theoretical biologist Robert Rosen coined the expression *"Anticipatory Systems"* for these behaviours of anticipation that are observed at all levels of organization of living systems. But biologists still continue to try to explain life using classical causality, such as predictive models or processes of natural selection. But, when we study the anticipatory behaviour of biological molecules, this cannot be explained as the result of natural selection, because we are considering a level upstream of the processes of natural selection, and cannot be the result of predictive models, because molecules are not equipped with cognitive systems capable of producing such models.

The hypothesis of the theory of syntropy is that retrocausality acts at all levels of life and when working with living systems it is possible to perform experiments that demonstrate the existence of retrocausality.

This was the main hypothesis behind Antonella Vannini's PhD dissertation and experiments.

Q: Let us introduce Antonella?

UDC: Antonella Vannini is my wife. I met her on January 7, 2001. At the time, my work on syntropy was blocked. Antonella told me that she had abandoned university, since she had to work, and that her dream was to go back again to university. Two days later we went out. It was a beautiful evening with a full moon eclipse. The day after 10:01:01, January 10, 2001, we engaged. We married nine months later, the same date, but upside down, 10:10:01, October 10, 2001. As a gift I gave Antonella the possibility to go back to university. I told her to choose listening to her heart and she chose cognitive psychology. Initially Antonella was not interested in syntropy, but working on her first thesis she encountered the equation with the dual energy solution and after a short time her thesis was titled: *"Entropy and Syntropy. From mechanical to life causation."* It was published in the NeuroQuantology Journal and it is now available at www.amazon.com/dp/1520783442 . After her bachelor's degree, she continued developing the topic of Syntropy in her master degree thesis, her PhD dissertation and in the dissertation for the Ericksonian school in hypnosis and psychotherapy. For the PhD in cognitive psychology Antonella conducted four experiments in order to test the retrocausal hypothesis that stems from the syntropy theory, according to which the parameters of the autonomic nervous systems, that supports life functions, must show pre-stimuli activations. More precisely skin conductance and heart rate should response BEFORE stimuli since the autonomic nervous system supports life functions acquiring syntropic energy which propagates backward-in-time. In the scientific literature some researchers had already found this strange pre-stimuli activation of the autonomic parameters, but there was no theory capable of explaining the rational of this strange effect. Antonella developed an experimental design which allows to observe a strong anticipatory effect of the heart rates. Results showed that the heart reacts before stimuli with emotional content.

Q: Can you provide an example?

UDC: I will now describe the experimental design devised by Antonella. A person was asked to sit in front of a computer monitor and with a heart rate detection strap applied to his/her chest. The trial consisted of three phases, in the first phase colours were presented full screen, such as the colour blue, green, red and yellow. Each colour remained on the screen for exactly 4 seconds. In the second phase the four colours were presented together as colour bars and the person had to try to guess the colour that the computer would have selected randomly in the third and final phase. In the last phase, that is, after the person expressed his guess for one of the colours, the computer started a random algorithm that led to select one of the four colours. At this point the selected colour was shown on the computer screen.

Phase 1 Presentation of stimuli and measurement of heart rate				Phase 2 Choice	Phase 3 Random selection
Blue	Green	Red	Yellow	Blue/Green/Red/Yellow	Red
					Target
4 seconds	4 seconds	4 seconds	4 seconds		

Each subject repeated the trial for 100 times. What the results show is that in the first phase the heart rates differ depending on the colour that the computer will select, in an unpredictable way, in the last phase (target colour). This activation is independent from the guess made by the subject in the second phase.

Q: More precisely?

UDC: For example, in some subjects the heart rate increases, in the first phase, when the computer will select the red colour as the target colour in the third phase. Each subject shows a different anticipatory heart rate configuration. The differences among target colours, in the activation of the heart rate within each individual, is highly significant. Each subject produces a specific pattern in response to what the computer will select 15 seconds later, in the third phase. So not a split of a second before, but a big activation well before. This activation is strong, both from a quantitative point of view, approximately two heartbeats of difference, and from a statistical point of view.

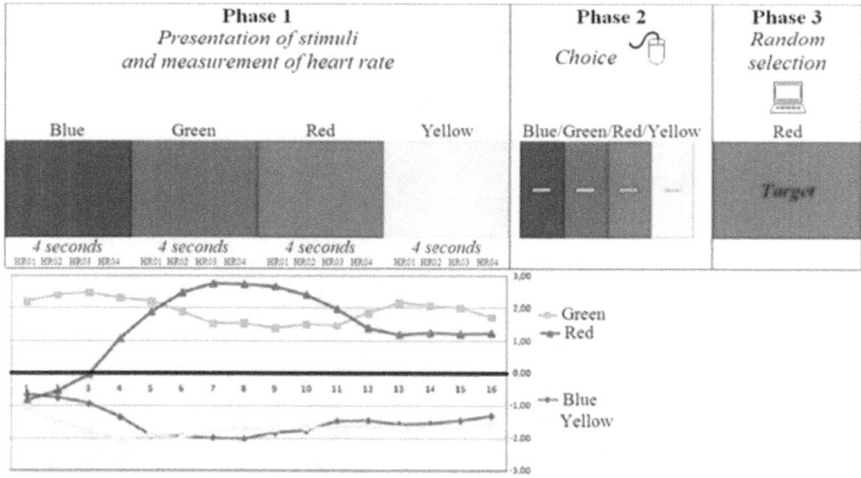

We can here see that the pre-activations of the heart rate, in phase one, in concomitance with the target colour which the computer selects in phase 3, differ from the base value, the zero line. In the absence of a retrocausal effect, lines should vary around the base value, the zero line. But the average heart rate values of the 100 trials, when associated to the target colour, differ significantly from the baseline.

Although the heart reacts in advance, at the cognitive level no advanced reaction was detectable. People guessed in phase 2 randomly. Consequently, a dissociation between the brain and the heart seems to take place. What the heart knows is not available for the brain. The heart already knows in advance what the computer will select, but the brain shows no knowledge about it.

Q: Are we talking about spontaneous but not conscious reactions?

UDC: In psychology we speak of implicit and explicit knowledge. The knowledge of the heart is implicit, that of the brain is explicit. Although we already know at the implicit level what the computer will select, at the explicit level this knowledge is not accessible.

When Antonella's positive results confirmed the scientific validity of the theory of syntropy, which had been relegated within philosophy, the reactions became violent. The professors, quantum physicists and cognitive psychologists, started attacking Antonella: *"This effect is impossible, it cannot exist, we are not going to look at the data!"*, *"You are a fraud, you invented the data!"*, *"You should be expelled from the academia!"*. They rejected the idea to replicate the experiments. As in the days of Galileo, where authorities refused to look into the telescope, now the authorities refused to see the data and analyse them independently. Attacks worsened and were at the personal level. One of the major professors of Quantum Mechanics went to the extent of suggesting that the result could be caused by a magic interaction between expectations of the subject and the electronic of the computer, which would determine the outcome of the random selection of the colour in phase 3. This was considered to be more acceptable. Antonella devised a series of controls. For example, after the computer had selected the target a second random procedure was used to determine whether to show or not the target on the computer screen. The anticipatory effect was visible in the data only when the computer displayed the selected target colour and not when it was not displayed. If the effect had been caused by an interaction between expectations and electronics determining the selection of the target colour according to forward-in-time causality (although magic), the effect would show either when the computer shows the target colour, and when is does not show it. Instead, the effect was visible only when the selected colour was shown to the subject. Consequently forward-in-time explanations were not possible.

Fantappiè had been accused of failing to produce any experimental evidence. When Antonella produced experimental evidences the reactions were of personal and direct attack. It was not acceptable that someone could question the law of cause and effect. CAUSES MUST ALWAYS PRECEDE THEIR EFFECTS. And this dogma could not be questioned. Antonella was under attack. Instead of evaluating the results and data of her experiments, the academia was trying to force Antonella to renounce to the dissertation discrediting her.

Meanwhile, the Dean of the Faculty of Engineering and Applied Sciences of the Princeton University, Robert Jahn, who had followed one of Antonella's presentations in a conference held in Norway, became enthusiastic of the experiments and results. Antonella translated her dissertation into English and sent it to Robert Jahn. Jahn had conducted similar experiments. They started during the Vietnam war when the president of McDonald Douglas asked Jahn, who was considered one of the leading scientists in the United States and was a Nobel laureate candidate, to study the anomalies that fighter jets showed in the electronic during the moments of combat. Jahn was a sceptic, but coincidentally a young student asked him to conduct experiments on the anomalous interaction between emotions and electronics. Jahn, sure that the experiments would have not led to any positive result, accepted since it was a good exercise for a dissertation. Results were positive and easy to replicate, and showed that emotions interact with electronics. Therefore, during combat the electronic can malfunction because of the strong emotional stress of the pilot. Jahn, together with Brenda Dunne, founded the PEAR laboratory (Princeton Engineering Anomalies Reasearch Laboratory). Experiments have been conducted for over thirty years and show, beyond any possible doubt, that there is a strong interaction between emotions and electronics. Moreover, they show a stronger effect when the experiment is devised in a retrocausal way. During combat pilots undergo extreme emotional stress, since they are close to death, and these emotions interact with the electronics. Shielding this anomalous interactions was studied and results were used in the military field and by NASA.

Jahn appreciated Antonella'a work and wrote a letter asking her to publish a book with ICRL (International Consciousness Research Laboratories). This book is now available with the title "*Syntropy, the Spirit of Love*": www.amazon.com/dp/1936033178 .

The experiments conducted by Antonella are simple to replicate. Antonella was a PhD student without a scholarship, the university did not provide equipments or funding. Everything, heart rate monitors and computers, were self-financed. The academia continued to reject the possibility that causality works differently and also the PEAR lab came under attack. Despite the total absence of support by the academia, I consider these experiments among the most interesting and important experiments which have been conducted in Italy in the last years.

Q: Did Jahn and his equip know about syntropy and Fantappiè's work?

UDC: The contact was established in 2007. We had been invited to give talks in Norway where we presented the theory of syntropy. The theory of syntropy is still poorly understood. It was impossible to publish the results of the experiments on mainstream scientific journals. Any result that challenges the law of cause and effect was rejected, even if supported by experimental results which are easy to replicate and control.

Q: Tell me more about this contact ...

UDC: Antonella searched for people who were conducting similar studies. She found Robert Jahn and Brenda Dunne, but also Dean Radin, Senior Scientist at the Institute of Noetic Sciences in California. With Jahn and Brenda Dunne in particular we exchanged emails and received guidance. We assessed different experimental designs in order to choose that which seemed more appropriate for the syntropy hypothesis. Jahn sent Antonella a letter inviting her to publish with ICRL. Antonella showed this letter to one of the professors of the Faculty of Psychology who had always discredited her work and the syntropy hypothesis. A couple of days later, this professor wrote to the Dean of the Faculty of Psychology and to the director of the PhD School, accusing Antonella of using his ideas, data and results, and asking to banish her from the university and from the PhD school. The Dean and the director of the PhD school, and all the other professors who had been involved in this dispute, were against Antonella, her experiments and the theory of syntropy, and were puzzled when this professor attributed to himself the experiments, showing such a strong interest for the results.

For several months Antonella was in the centre of a hurricane, a huge conflict. But coincidences turned this conflict into the recognition of her work. When the moment came and she had to defend her dissertation in front of the national commission, Antonella was left alone. No one was there, her tutors were terrified and did not show up. All those who had previously attacked her did not show. Everyone was afraid.

Antonella questioned the topic of causality, the untouchable DOGMA of the law of cause and effect. Whoever advocates a different type of causality knows that he will be treated as an heretic, an enemy of the academia, and marginalized. Few people have the courage to support the hypothesis that causality works differently.

Q: A dogmatic religion?

UDC: When Fantappiè suggested that he could see the properties of life in backward-in-time causality, he was fiercely censored. When Robert Jahn started asserting that causality works differently he was expelled from the academia, but the Princeton University had to re-assign him the post. Jahn tells that the same academics that in public attacked him, in private told him that they agreed with him, but that they could not support him, otherwise they risked their position and funds.

Q: This reminds me of Hahnemann and homeopathy.

UDC: This is the reason of this interview. Fantappiè had repeatedly shown interest for homeopathy as he could interpret its effects according to retrocausality. Everyone had tried to explain homeopathy according to classical causality, even the hypothesis of the memory of water, although original, tries to explain homeopathy according to classical causality. What I want to say is that we must have the courage to say that living systems are supercausal systems, driven mainly by causes that emanate from the future.

Q: When you talk about retrocausality you talk also about a change in paradigm.

UDC: Yes. When we say that there is an additional type of causality, which flows backward-in-time, we are stating the existence of a new paradigm. Currently the mechanistic paradigm dominates and billions are spent to keep together this paradigm. The Higgs boson provides an example. Classical causality is governed by entropy and it is diverging. It does not account for converging forces, such as gravity. What causes gravity? Why bodies attract? The Higgs boson tries to provide an answer, but it is extremely contradictory and uses a complex and questionable mathematics. It is the cause of converging forces, provided by the mechanistic paradigm, which most people have accepted although the statistical significance was very limited. The theory of syntropy explains gravity and converging forces as the manifestation of attractors (i.e. backward-in-time causality), and suggests that gravity should propagate instantaneously, that atoms vibrate very quickly from diverging to converging states. Billions are spent to keep standing the standard model of particles, on which the mechanistic paradigm is based, but people working on retrocausality and the backward-in-time solution are denied any funding.

The paradigm shift towards supercausality has countless implications. In statistics and scientific methodology, which is the field in which I provide my work, it implies the shift from the methodology of differences, which is at the basis of the experimental method, to the methodology of concomitant variations. The methodology of concomitant variations was described in 1843 by the economist and philosopher John Stuart Mill. In order to scientifically study causality the method of differences can be coupled with the method of concomitant variations. The methodology of differences starts with two similar groups, a treatment (or cause) is given, to the experimental group and not to the control group. Differences between the two groups can be attributed only to the treatment.

Differences can study only a few variables at a time and require quantitative and objective measurements, distributed in a Gaussian way. The methodology of concomitant variations, instead, allows to study an unlimited number of quantitative and quantitative variables together. Since syntropy manifests itself mainly in the form of qualitative and subjective experiences, the methodology of concomitant variations is particularly important when studying living systems. The method of differences cannot handle qualitative and subjective information. It has therefore brought to believe that the syntropic and invisible side of reality is by definition outside of science and can be accessed only through subjective experiences and religion. In statistics techniques can be grouped according to the methodology of differences, such as ANOVA and Student's t, and techniques based on the methodology of concomitant variations, such as Chi-square and contingencies tables. The methodology of concomitant variations does not imply a causal direction and can therefore study both forward and backward-in-time causality.

Q: So if I grabbed it correctly ... statistics already provides tools which allow to work correctly within the new paradigm.

UDC: Yes, the methodology of concomitant variations is already here, in the form of statistical techniques that can be used with great ease. We have published the book *"The Methodology of Concomitant Variations"* www.amazon.com/dp/1520326637 and provide free statistical software through our website www.sintropia.it . Until the late sixties the use of computers was prohibitive. Researchers were forced to use statistical techniques that could be calculated by hand. This led to the methodology of differences and the experimental method. Now we are ready for the methodology of concomitant variations and the shift to the supercausal paradigm. The tools are ready.

Obviously there are big economic and political interests. The pharmaceutical industries based on the mechanistic paradigm oppose this shift of paradigm. The new paradigm inevitably leads to a new type of medicine, such as homeopathic or natural medicines based on the concept of life energy. Furthermore the methodology of differences permits to manipulate the results and this is frequently done, whereas the methodology of concomitant variations does not allow for manipulation of the results. Any manipulation would result in visible incoherent data.

The methodology of concomitant variations is robust, easy, difficult to manipulate, but scientific journals which are mainly financed by the pharmaceutical industries, require data analyses that use the old methodology of differences. Studies show that over 80% of the results published in the major scientific journals using the methodology of differences, cannot be replicated. Just by changing mean values or removing outliers it is possible to see effects that are inexistent. This is often done in order to attend a scientific conference, to receive grants or publish in a scientific journal. A science based on false results has become the norm and drugs with no therapeutic effect are now sold. The manipulation of results is rather impossible when using the method of concomitant variations. This methodology opens the doors to the new supercausal paradigm.

There is another very important point that we need to address and it is that of water.

Syntropy is available at the quantum level, while entropy is the law which governs the macroscopic world in which we live. Then, how does life draw syntropy from the quantum world?

In 1925 the physicist Wolfgang Pauli discovered in water molecules the hydrogen bond or hydrogen bridge. Hydrogen atoms are located in an intermediate position between the sub-atomic level, quantum, and the molecular level of the macrocosm, allowing the flow of syntropy from the micro to the macro.

Q: But why water?

UDC: The water molecule is made of oxygen and hydrogen. When water molecules bind, hydrogen atoms are in a state between quantum and the macrocosm level. A limbo between both these levels.

The hydrogen bonding acquires syntropy from the quantum level. Since syntropy is converging energy, water has cohesive properties and shows binding forces which are ten times more powerful than the van der Waals forces that hold together other liquids. Because of these significant cohesive forces, water manifests anomalous properties. For example, when it freezes it expands, it becomes less dense and floats; when other liquids solidify they contract, become more dense, heavy and sink. The singularity of water lies almost entirely in these powerful cohesive forces, typical of the law of syntropy. The other molecules that form hydrogen bonds, such as ammonia, do not reach these high cohesive properties and therefore cannot construct networks and wide structures in space as it is the case for water. Hydrogen bonds allow syntropy to flow from the micro to the macro, from the quantum to the macrocosm, making water molecule essential for life. Water is, ultimately, the lymph of life, that supplies living organisms with syntropy. If life is ever to start on another planet, certainly water should be present. Water is essential for the creation and evolution of any biological structure.

Based on these considerations, in February 2011 I wrote with Antonella a commentary in the Journal of Cosmology. Richard Hoover of NASA's Marshall Space Flight Center, discovered micro fossils of cyanobacteria in meteorites of comets. The theory of syntropy states that life is a general law of the universe, that is manifested in the presence of water. A characteristic of comets is to be rich in ice which in the vicinity of the Sun melts and becomes water. In our review we have therefore suggested that the theory of syntropy provides an explanation for the formation of living organisms, even in extreme situations, such as those that are found on comets, and that the discovery of micro fossils by Richard Hoover is consistent with syntropy.

To better understand the implications of the hydrogen bond it is important to clarify the three types of time that the theory of syntropy posits:

1. *Causal time* is expected in diverging systems, such as our expanding Universe, and it is governed by the forward-in-time solution of the equations. In diverging systems entropy prevails, causes always precede effects and time flows forward, from the past to the future. The law of Entropy forbids retrocausality. It is therefore not possible to see light waves that go backward-in-time or receive radio signals before they are transmitted.
2. *Retrocausal time* is expected in converging systems, as it is the case of black-holes. Retrocausal time is governed by the backward-in-time solution of the equations. In converging systems retrocausality prevails, effects always precede causes and time flows backwards, from the future to the past. In these systems it is impossible to see light coming out from black holes since energy moves backward-in-time and the forward-in-time flow is impossible.
3. *Supercausal time* characterizes systems in which diverging and converging forces are balanced. An example is provided by atoms, the quantum level of matter. In these systems, causality and retrocausality coexist and time is unitary: past, present and future coincide.

This classification of time was already present in Greece in the form of: Kronos, Kairos and Aion.

- *Kronos* describes sequential time, which is familiar to us, the forward-in-time solutions of the equations: absolute moments that flow from the past to future.
- *Kairos* describes retrocausal time, the backward-in-time solution of the equations. According to Pythagoras, Kairos is at the basis of intuitions and the ability to anticipate the future and to choose advantageously.
- *Aion* describes supercausal time in which past, present and future coexist. This is the time of the quantum world, the sub-atomic world.

Water molecules allow life to acquire syntropy from the quantum level and to connect to a unitary time where past, present and future coexist.

D: This is fantastic! It sounds like one of those fantasy movies where water works as a portal, a door between different worlds.

UDC: between two different realms. Water has properties which are completely different from all the other liquids and allows causality to operate in a way which is different from classical forward-in-time causality.

Q: Can you provide an example?

UDC: The properties of water are symmetrical with respect to other liquids. For example, it can absorb enormous amounts of heat, exactly as expected according to syntropy. This peculiarity of water explains why it is used in cooling systems. The ability of water to absorb heat is incredible, the thermal properties of water show how syntropy absorbs energy. Another example: ice is less dense than water and therefore floats. All other molecules are more dense in their solid form, since when they solidify they contract, they become more dense and heavy and sink. With water just the opposite happens, water is more dense.

Water solidifies starting from the top. Other liquids solidify starting from below, since heat moves up towards the surface. The liquid in the lower part is therefore the first to reach the solidification temperature, and for this reason liquids solidify from the bottom. Again, in order to increase water temperature more heat is needed than that which is required for other liquids. The singularity of water lies almost entirely in its attractive, cohesive and absorption properties that are typical of syntropy. Given the importance that water plays in providing syntropy, living systems are made mostly of water. We humans are 70% made of water. Water is not a neutral molecule, but it is a molecule that can have huge effects on life. In order to activate these properties it is necessary to act according to retrocausality, the logic of syntropy, which is symmetrical to classic causality. For example, if we want to have a strong effect, instead of increasing the active substance, we need to dilute it. This is precisely what we see in Homeopathy and this is the reason why Fantappiè became interested in Homeopathy.

Q: Prof. Negro who was the dean of the Italian Homeopathy met Fantappiè several times. Fantappiè could see in Homeopathy a proof of his theory of syntropy.

UDC: Fantappiè was looking for a way to test his theory, but the experimental method requires that causes precede effects and does not allow to study retrocausal effects. On the contrary homeopathy is constantly working with retrocausality and the anomaly of homeopathy is precisely due to this, namely, that causality is reversed and somehow Fantappiè saw homeopathy as a confirmation of his theory of syntropy. Fantappiè found himself in a paradoxical situation. The theory of syntropy stems from the fundamental equations of physics, but the experimental validation of this theory seems possible only when studying living systems and, therefore, also in the field of medicine.

Q: I find this singular.

UDC: Feynman and Wheeler, both Nobel laureates in physics, came to the conclusion that when experiments are carried in physics the retrocausal effect cannot be distinguished from classical forward-in-time causality. For example, it is impossible to tell if a positron moves backward or forward-in-time. The equations say that it moves backward-in-time, however, if it moves backward or forward the results are the same, and consequently experiments cannot distinguish between causality and retrocausality. This difficulty prevents experimental tests in physics. Instead in life sciences exactly the opposite happens. The theory of syntropy puts physics in a subordinate position to life sciences.

Q: I have a profane curiosity, at this point. The question may seem trivial to you or out of context. My Homeopathy professor (I refer to dr. Spinedi) in a conference in Verona in 2013, after the presentation of some case studies, received the praise of Fritjof Capra, who enthusiastically told him that this is the new medicine! But is the new physics ready to accept retrocausality?

UDC: I met Fritjof Capra and I know his work. However Fritjof Capra, like many other physicists who speak about the new physics, has not had the courage to embrace the topic of retrocausality. So on the one hand he talks of the crisis of the mechanistic paradigm, but on the other hand he does not have the courage to really go beyond the mechanistic paradigm.

Q: That was indeed my question. I now rephrase it: how do the new physicists see retrocausality? It seems to me that the new physicists should have sympathy and understanding for retrocausality and Homeopathy.

UDC: Many new physics state that the mechanistic paradigm is in a crisis, but generally speaking they are not suggesting any way out. Those very few who have the audacity and courage to make the crossing to supercausality and retrocausality are attacked, discredited and excluded from grants and from the academia. There is a violent censorship. Those who have done the crossing to supercausality say that the price they had to pay is so high that they often advise others not to do it! Many prefer to remain in the classical mainstream science, and compromise. With me and Antonella it is different. We have the opportunity to talk openly about retrocausality and supercausality since we decided to stay out of the academic world. We are able to make a living without having to compromise.

The mechanistic paradigm is governed by the law of entropy that leads to increase disorder, dissipation and conflicts and according to the syntropy theory, the mounting crisis of the Western societies is nothing else than the manifestation of entropy. In order to come out from this crisis the transition to the supercausal paradigm is required. But physics has become similar to a medieval church, which burns at stake the heretics. As in the days of Giordano Bruno. In life sciences and especially in economics, which is probably the discipline mostly affected by the crisis, the mechanistic paradigm no longer works. The need for the transition is broadly felt. In physics this need is not felt. Physicists feel content with the mechanistic paradigm which provides them a central role. I think that the transition will start in economics and subsequently in biology, psychology and medicine. But, what I expect is that biologists, doctors, psychologists and economists will provide the experimental proof to the new paradigm. Life sciences will not be subordinate to physicists, but physics will have to listen to biologists, psychologists and economists and who will provide the experimental validation of syntropy. A new physics extended to the laws of life. Just to say, we were contacted recently by physicists of the Berkeley University. They read our articles and essays. One of them told us that she could not sleep all night for the incredible implications that she could see in our works. Many physicists know that it is time to change paradigm, but in physics it is very difficult, whereas in life sciences it seems easier.

Q: Can you give a reason for this?

UDC: My tutor Vittorio Castellano used to associate the difference between the old and new paradigm to the difference between mathematics and statistics. Mathematics is deterministic. Functions provide always only one result. When dealing with square roots, which have always a positive and negative solution, in order to maintain determinism, it has been arbitrary decided that only the positive result is taken into account. On the contrary statistic is non-deterministic. Mathematics is at the foundation of the mechanistic paradigm, whereas statistics is required in life sciences where the supercausal paradigm is more evident. The focus on mathematics (and also on parametric statistics, i.e. mathematical statistics) has limited physics to the old paradigm.

Q: What about Hahnemann and vital energy?

UDC: According to syntropy, vital energy is energy which diverges backward-in-time. But physicists have rejected this backward-in-time energy, since it questions the law of cause and effect. The backward-in-time energy requires a new language and formalism. We need to shift to non-parametric statistics and the implications are huge not only in the field of economics, where mathematics has caused enormous disasters, but also in biology, psychology and medicine. Darwinism provides an example. This approach works well within microevolution, that is when species adapt to environments by reducing their genetic information, but does not work when it comes to macroevolution, that is when there is an increase in complexity. For example, let us consider one of the simplest increases in complexity: the formation of a protein starting from amino acids. The simplest protein is composed of about 90 amino acids. The possibility that amino acids combine in the right sequence giving place to the simplest protein is, according to combinatorial science, less than one over a number followed by 600 zeros. Elsasser in the paper *A causal phenomena in physics and biology: A case for reconstruction*, published in 1969 in the American Scientist (vol. 57, pp. 502-16) shows that in the 13-15 billion years of our Universe a maximum of 10^{106} simple events (at the nanosecond level) have taken place. Consequently, any event which requires a combinatory value greater than 10^{106} simply cannot apply to our physical Universe. Since 10^{600} (one followed by 600 zeroes) is greater than all the combinations which have taken place since the Big Bang, the possibility of the spontaneous formation of the simplest protein is nil. Elsasser's results show that the notion of mechanical causation in biology is devoid of logical underpinning and that its use is metaphorical at best. A real danger exists that the use of this metaphor can too easily divert one's attention in the wrong direction. In practice, considering all the history of the Universe and all the spontaneous combinations, it is impossible that a single protein may form just by chance. Furthermore, when this protein would eventually come out by chance, it would be immediately destroyed by entropy. So, adhering to the mechanistic paradigm the formation of life is simply impossible, and chance does not provide an explanation. Even more inexplicable is the formation of cells, organisms and individuals. Without speaking of consciousness and feelings.

Syntropy attributes life properties to attractors which operate from the quantum level through water. Each attractor provides information, but it also receives information, selects that which is advantageous for life and redistributes it. Attractors progressively grow in complexity and since they depend on the properties of the backward-in-time energy solutions, which allow for entanglement and non-local instantaneous correlations, their in-formation can be transferred and received everywhere in the Universe. Attractors are one of the fundamental concepts introduced by the theory of syntropy. They act from the quantum level and guide towards a specific designs. Attractors grow in complexity, similarly to forward-in-time energy which coalesces thanks to cohesive forces such as gravity, backward-in-time energy coalesces thanks to entropy. The physical visible universe is organized into galaxies, solar systems, planets, etc., the invisible world is organized in a hierarchy of attractors which specialize and guide towards specific forms and designs. Life attractors require water to organize and manifest. In the absence of water the activation of these attractors is impossible. Syntropy leads to the conclusion that life is a manifestation of the interaction between the quantum and the macro levels through water. When water is not present life is impossible. Thus in the presence of water life is being created continuously. Life is caused by complex attractors that guide towards specific designs. DNA are antennas which link to these complex attractors. Information is not stored in genes but outside in the attractors. Specific attractors exists for each species. Darwinian theory based on trial and errors and natural selection can explain microevolution, whereas macroevolution is an intelligent process which can be explained by the action of attractors. Intelligent information is stored in the attractors and constantly acts from the quantum level, guiding evolution.

Q: You have used the word "attractors", can you tell us more about it?

UDC: When it comes to classical causality we talk about causes, when we talk about retrocausality we deal with attractors. In 1963 the meteorologist Edward Lorenz discovered the existence of attractors which make systems sensitive, at every point, to small changes. For example, studying at the computer a simple meteorological model, he realized that with a small change in the initial conditions a *"chaotic state"* can amplify making any prediction impossible. By analysing this system that behaves so unpredictably, Lorenz found the existence of an attractor which is now named *"the chaotic attractor of Lorenz."* This attractor allows microscopic perturbations to be enormously amplified and interfere with the macroscopic behaviour of the system. Lorenz himself described this situation with the famous words: *"The flap of a butterfly's wings in the Amazon can cause a hurricane in the United States."* In meteorology, as well as in other disciplines that deal with water, such as life sciences, one continually encounters attractors. Attractors are observed and described, but scientists do not know what causes them. In other words, they observe the effect of syntropy (attractors), but do not speak of syntropy. Science is still tied to the mechanistic paradigm, and attractors are observed and described, but they are still a mystery. All what is converging is a mystery for the old paradigm. Not least the force of gravity.

The constant flow of information from the past, in the form of memories and experiences, and the in-formation that comes from the future, in the form of emotions that attract us toward a specific direction, constantly show bifurcations, and we need to choose which one we want to follow. Do we choose the head or the heart? This constant state of choice is at the basis of free will and chaotic dynamics. In other words, when causality and retrocausality interact, the system becomes chaotic and non-deterministic. The discovery of attractors gave rise to the science of chaos.

Entropy tends to level effects, syntropy tends to amplify effects. A field where the interaction between causality and retrocausality becomes visible is that of fractal geometry. The term fractal was coined in 1975 by Benoît Mandelbrot, and it is derived from the Latin word fractus (broken). Fractals appear in chaos theory and are obtained by inserting geometric attractors in the form of limits to which the system tends. For example, if we repeat the square root of a number greater than zero, but lower than one, the result will tend to one, but it will never reach it. Number one is the attractor. Similarly, if we continue to square a number greater than one the result will tend to infinity and if we continue to square a number less than one, the result will tend to zero. Fractal figures are obtained when attractors are used.

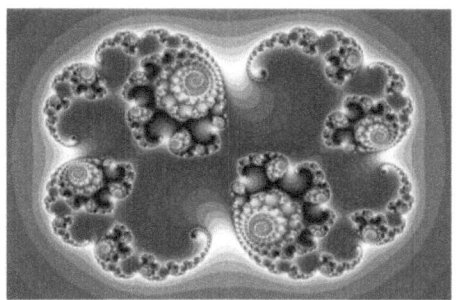 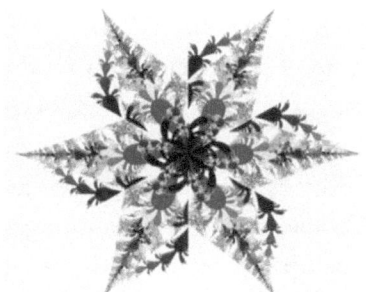

Examples of fractal images taken from Wikipedia

Mandelbrot showed that these figures are complex, but at the same time ordered. Fractal geometry has captivated many researchers because of their similarity with the organization of living systems. The coronary arteries and veins have fractal ramifications. The main vessels branch into a series of smaller vessels that, in turn, branch out in vessels of even more reduced calibre. These fractal structures seem to have a vital role in the mechanics of contraction and in the conduct of excitatory electrical stimulation: the spectral analysis of the heart rate shows that the normal beat is characterized by a broad spectrum that resembles chaotic fractal patterns. Also neurons have a structure similar to fractals, with asymmetric ramifications (dendrites) associated with cell bodies, which at a slightly higher magnification show similar ramifications. Lungs resemble fractals. Bronchi and bronchioles form a tree with multiple ramifications, whose configuration looks alike at high and low magnification. By measuring the diameters of different orders of branching, it was found that the bronchial tree can be described by fractal geometry. Fractal geometry suggests that the organization and evolution of living systems (tissues, nervous systems, living organisms and species) are driven by attractors that guide the living system thanks to the retrocausal properties of syntropy.

Another field in which attractors are studied are vortices. Vortices are caused by attractors, for example by gravity. In vortices the famous "golden ratio" is always found. Leonardo of Pisa wrote in 1202 the book "*Liber Abaci*" (or "The Book of Calculation") under the pen-name "Fibonacci." This work proved a significant contribution to the history of mathematics because it introduced the use of Arabic numerals into Europe, which eventually replaced Roman numerals. Fibonacci described a sequence of numbers that is known as Fibonacci Numbers, although this sequence had already been used in Sanskrit poetry as early as 450 BC. Fibonacci called this sequence Modus Indorum (method of the Indians), and applied it to problems involving the growth of a population of rabbits based on idealized assumptions. The solution turned out to be a sequence of numbers that was the sum of the two previous numbers. The ratio between the numbers in a Fibonacci sequence (1.618034) is called the Golden Ratio, or Golden Section, and can be found throughout nature.

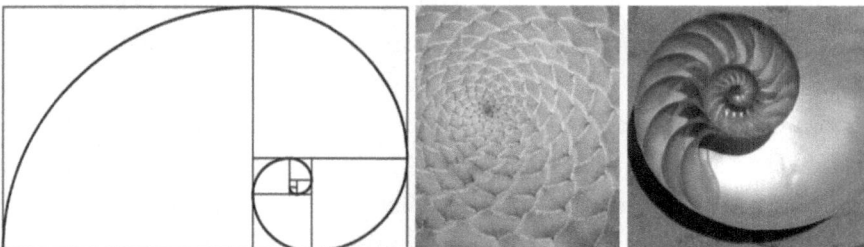

Examples of Fibonacci sequences

Fractal geometry and the spiral shape of the Golden Ratio reproduce some of the most important structures of living systems, and many researchers believe that life follows these two principles: the leaf arrangement in plants, the pattern of the florets of a flower, grains of wheat, the growth of corals, a hive of bees, the form of the brain and neurons, as well as the lungs. Fibonacci numbers appear to be applicable to the growth of every living thing.

Attractors do not cancel entropy, but they establish a bridge between entropy and syntropy and provide proportions that were already known in antiquity. What I find interesting is the interdisciplinary of this approach. The theory of syntropy merges together not only physics and biology, but all disciplines, from sciences to arts and spirituality. Syntropy can be found in all the aspects of reality like a thread that connects everything. Everything seems to result from the continuous interaction between diverging and converging forces. Living systems tend to converge towards the attractor, and when they diverge suffering and crises are the outcome.

Q: Do you think that syntropy may have socio-economic, political and even international implications?

UDC: Yes I believe that the crisis is a consequence of the mechanistic paradigm and in order to solve it we need to shift to the new supercausal and syntropic paradigm. Just an example, with Antonella we have hold seminars for the PhD School in Management at the University of Rome La Sapienza. Economists make the distinction between problem solving and decision making. Decision making is strategic, future-oriented. Case studies show that effective decision making is based on intuitions and guided by the heart. How can we account for this in science? Syntropy connects intuitions to aims and attractors. The information coming from the past is typically handled by the brain, is based on memory, experiences, facts, but it is not oriented, whereas information coming from the future, is based on feelings that attract towards a specific direction. We feel to be attracted towards a specific aim. Free will arises from the constant state of choice between what our past experiences tell and where our feelings attract us. We are constantly in front of these bifurcations and we are forced to choose. We must choose between the head and the heart. But, when decisions are important we need to follow the intuitive side. The head is useful in problem solving, based on experience. The heart and intuitions are necessary in decision-making. The neurophysiologist Antonio Damasio discovered that people with decision making deficits have poor or little perception of their emotional feelings. This deficiency is common among those who have lesions in the frontal lobe of the brain, or that use substances such as alcohol and heroin that "anesthetize" the feelings of the heart. However, these people show intact cognitive functions. Short and long term memory, working memory, attention, perception, language, logic, arithmetic, intelligence, learning, knowledge of the elements of the problem to which is asked to make the decision and the integrity of the system of values are all intact. They respond normally to the majority of the tests and their cognitive functions are normal; despite this, they are not able to decide in an appropriate manner for all that concerns their future. This leads to a dissociation between the ability to solve problems and the ability to decide. Damasio found that decision-making deficits are always accompanied by alterations in the ability to feel, whereas cognitive abilities are intact. When feelings are impaired we observe the inability to plan for the future, the inability to make a program for the hours to come, the confusion with respect to priorities and lack of insight. Individuals with decision making deficit are characterized by knowledge but not by feeling. Damasio shows that the feelings which are useful in decision-making are primarily those of the heart, in the form of the acceleration of the heartbeat, followed by those of the lungs, in the form of the contraction of breath, intestines and muscles. These feelings are used in decision-making and help to build advantageous strategies. Damasio notes that emotions help to direct and guide our decisions and lead to the appropriate place of a space in which decision-making can work well without the tools of logic. Damasio's results suggest that there is a system driven by emotions and feelings that is oriented toward the future, and that this system is at the basis of decision-making. When a person loses its contact with emotions and feelings, the future-oriented drive is lost and it becomes difficult to choose advantageously. Feelings act like the needle of a compass that points in the direction which is most advantageous. We need to learn to read this compass of the heart. Our excessive focus on the brain has made us unaware of this compass.

D: Which political approach do you consider syntropic?

UDC: I believe that all parties can benefit from the syntropic vision of life and society. Syntropy is horizontal and is neither right nor left. It rather tends to harmonize opposite positions. Furthermore, political organizations, associations or movements generate power struggles. This is antithetical to the whole message of syntropy, which is based on cooperation and convergence. Syntropy leads to envision a mixture between direct democracy and meritocracy. Western representative democracy is the product of the industrial age and the mechanistic paradigm, profoundly dysfunctional for nature and the happiness and wellbeing of people. In order to work on the theory of syntropy I had to stay away from the academic world and from politics. I had to prioritize my freedom of thought. This does not mean that syntropy cannot enter the academic or the political and business worlds. The theory of syntropy provides effective and costless solutions to problems that now seem mysterious. It clearly shows the way, it leads to effective and efficient strategies, and can therefore be useful for managers, as well as policy makers and statesmen. Syntropy can serve whoever is working for the promotion of life and the wellbeing of people and humanity.

Q: I was wondering which are the implications at the economic level.

UDC: The implications are simply enormous. The syntropy theory says that we always have to tend to *reduce entropy and increase syntropy*. The mechanistic paradigm, instead, constantly increases entropy and reduces syntropy and this is the cause of the crisis we are now witnessing. If we continue to think in a cause and effect manner entropy will continue to increase; conflicts, wars, the depletion of the environment and pollution will increase. We need to shift towards a future oriented vision of economics, where increasing syntropy and reducing entropy is synonymous of wealth, wellbeing and happiness.

Shifting towards the new supercausal and syntropic paradigm will be inevitable. The West is desperately trying to keep together the mechanistic paradigm, which is collapsing. It would rather go to a Third World War, instead of changing the paradigm. But the outcome would still be the change of paradigm. So, why not change the paradigm and avoid another destructive war? The change of paradigm can start from the bottom, from the people, and then propagate to economics, institutions and governments. This is the reason why I provide assistance to individuals who are trying to solve their existential crisis.

Obviously we all resist to change. But when we feel the attractor the direction becomes clear and it is difficult not to change. When we converge towards the attractor we feel wellbeing and warmth in the thorax area. When we diverge we feel void, pain, depression and anxiety. These feelings can be used as the needle of a compass, what I call the compass of the heart. We need to learn how to follow the indications of the compass of the heart and avoid external influences. Suffering informs us that we are on the wrong path, diverging from the attractor.

The *"Theory of Vital Needs"* stems from the constant struggle of life with entropy. For example, in order to counter entropy we must meet material conditions such as drinking, eating, shelter, and intangible conditions such as the need for meaning and the need for cohesion and love. When a vital need is met only partially an alarm bell is felt. For example, if we need to drink we feel thirsty, if we need to eat we feel hungry, if we need a shelter we feel cold or heat. The same applies to the intangible needs, for example if we need meaning we feel insignificant, useless and depressed. Depression is an alarm bell. It is similar to thirst and hunger and has the function to inform us that the vital need for meaning is not satisfied. Likewise anguish and anxiety inform us that the vital need for cohesion and love is not satisfied.

The theory of vital needs, adds to the well-known material needs for food, water, housing and sanitation, the immaterial needs for meaning and love. The end point of this theory is the theorem of love. The theorem of love solves the identity conflict between being and not being:

$$\frac{Syntropy}{Entropy} = 0$$

We are syntropy, we feel we exist. But when we compare ourselves to the outside universe which has inflated towards infinite thanks to entropy, we discover to be equal to zero. On one side we feel we exist, on the other side we are aware to be equal to zero. These two opposite considerations generate the identity conflict which was described by Shakespeare with the words: *"to be, or not to be: that is the question."*

The aim is to solve the identity conflict and this can be done only if we find a way to state our identity:

$$Syntropy = Syntropy$$

From a mathematical point of view this is possible only when we multiply the numerator of the identity conflict by Entropy:

$$\frac{Syntropy \times \cancel{Entropy}}{\cancel{Entropy}} = Syntropy$$

When we unite ourselves with the Universe (i.e. Entropy) the identity conflict and depression are solved and we experience the meaning of our life. Multiplications have the converging and cohesive properties of love. It is therefore possible to state that only through love we can solve depression and experience happiness. This is why this equation is named the *Theorem of Love*. The theorem of love shows that we can accomplish the transition from duality (I=0) to non-duality (I=I) and explains why anxiety (the lack of love) and depression (the lack of meaning) are perfectly correlated.

But, how can we love all the universe? If we carefully analyse the theorem of love it does not say that happiness is reached when we love all the universe, but it tells that love is the aim of life and that love and happiness coincide.

The theory of vital needs says that love gives meaning to our existence, and that only through love we can solve the conflict between being and non-being. Love causes an increase in the flow of syntropy and in the ability of the body to heal and regenerate. Healing is therefore strictly correlated to love.

Unfortunately, we are focused on material needs and try to explain anguish and depression solely as a result of a dysfunction of our chemical mediators. Psychiatry tries to cope with depression and anxiety by restoring the balance of our chemical mediators by means of drugs. What would you say if we were to solve starvation using drugs that eliminate the feeling of hunger? Would it seem a contradiction? After a while we would die. The same happens with anxiety and depression. We silence these feelings, but the real cause is not solved and continues to act worsening the suffering and the psychiatric symptomatology. Psychiatric diseases are spreading and psychology and psychiatry seem to be ineffective.

The supercausal paradigm says that the goal is to converge towards the attractor and that when this happens the flow of syntropy increases and we perceive feelings of warmth, love and wellbeing. Life fills with meaning and happiness. In order to converge we must not look for causes, but for attractors. We must look for what is invisible.

Q: Entropy goes towards the future and towards death, chaos and disorder and allopathic medicine goes in the same direction. Homeopathic medicine instead manifests a different tendency. During treatment patients can have flashes of past symptoms that were suppressed by allopathic drugs. Symptoms reappear in a backward-in-time sequence. It does not happen always, but often.

UDC: Allopathic medicine is based on the idea that causes must always precede their effects. This is governed by the law of entropy and leads to costs and increased public debt. The new paradigm offers solutions which are often counter intuitive. Let us see one. Duchenne, a type of muscular dystrophy that leads to death at an age that usually ranges between 18 and 24 years, is a genetic disease. Money goes therefore only to genetic studies, which have achieved little: patients continue to die between 18 and 24. In Denmark they have instead focused on the quality of life. Let us see how it works. In Italy, and most Western countries, the State spends approximately 10thousand euros per month for the home treatment and care of each Duchenne patient: money goes from the centre to the periphery: first to the Regions, then to the local health agencies, and then to foundations and cooperatives that provide care and treatment. In each step part of the money is lost and at the end the care which is provided is often minimal and often by unpaid volunteers. In Denmark the approach is reversed. Money is given directly in the hands of the Duchenne patient who chooses how to organize his care. Usually 3 or 4 care givers are hired full-time. They are well trained, taken from the free market, and not volunteers. If the Duchenne patient is not happy he can replace them at any moment. This results in a need for Training Schools. Professionals who feel the need to continuously update themselves. In short, in Denmark Duchenne patients live up to 40 years. A good quality life. Only by reversing the way how money flows and provide attention to the person, we shift from the mechanistic paradigm to a type of organization which is focused on attractors and life energies and creates a virtuous economy, which creates training schools, and which can be taxed at many different passages, enabling the government to recover all the money which was spent. Wellbeing and prosperity is created at no cost, just by reversing the way how we consider causality. Cost/benefit thinking is put on a side, the relevant role is given to feelings.

Q: It seems to me that this example provides a practical aspect of the application of syntropy on a specific problem, which like homeopathy also operates according to a simple and effective reversed causality.

UDC: Denmark has always rejected the EU welfare system and the Euro, since they have a different approach to how problems must be faced and solved. The EU is profoundly mechanistic and this is probably one of the major causes of the crisis of the Euro and of the Union.

Facts are showing that Danes are following a way by far more effective and efficient, and this provides a clue on how the theory of syntropy could be developed into a welfare system.

Reversing the way how we approach causality inevitably favours the transition from allopathic to homeopathic medicine.

All disciplines can be revised, by just reversing the way how we think to causality. This can be done in economics, social policies, architecture, decision making, medicine and psychology. The crisis of the Western World is due to the mechanistic paradigm which has come to an end.

Q: Really interesting.

UDC: Thank you!

2

RETROCAUSALITY

The fundamental equations describe the present as the meeting point of causes that act from the past (causality) and attractors that act from the future (retrocausality).

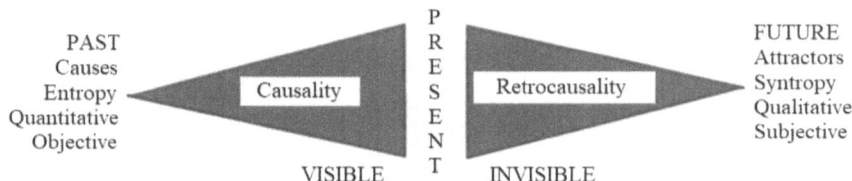

Let us see an example.

In 1803 Thomas Young showed, with the double slit experiment, that light propagates as waves:

The experiment I am about to talk about can be repeated with great ease, as long as the Sun is shining and with an instrumentation that is within everyone's reach
Thomas Young, 24 November 1803

Young's experiment was very simple. A ray of Sun goes through the slit of a screen that is indicated in the drawing below with S1, then reaches a second screen, S2, with two holes.

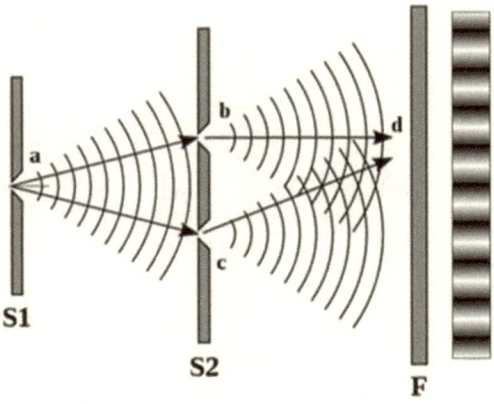

The light that goes through the two holes of the second screen finally ends up on the white screen F, where it creates a figure of lights and shadows. If the light had been made up of particles, two points of light should be observed, corresponding to the two holes in the second screen. Instead we observe a figure where dark and light bands alternate. Young explained this figure as a consequence of the fact that light propagates through the two holes like waves. These waves give rise to light bands in the points where they add up, that is, where there is constructive interference, while they give rise to dark bands in points where they do not add up, that is destructive interference.

Everything went well until the end of the nineteenth century when physicists found themselves in front of a paradox. Maxwell's equations led to predict that a black body, that is, an object that absorbs all the electromagnetic radiation, must emit ultraviolet frequencies with peaks of infinite power. Fortunately, this does not happen! This forecast, known as the ultraviolet catastrophe, has never been observed in nature.

The answer to this paradox was given on December 14th, 1900 by Max Planck. In an article that he presented to the German Physics Society, Planck suggested that energy does not propagate in the form of waves, but as multiples of fundamental units, packages that he called quanta. Quanta can be more or less small depending on the frequency of the vibration of the body. Under the quanta dimension energy does not propagate. This avoids the formation of infinite peaks of heat and resolved the paradox of the ultraviolet catastrophe.

In 1905 Einstein solved the paradox of the photoelectric effect describing light as composed of quanta, that is, particles rather than waves. The photoelectric effect consists in the fact that when the rays of light hit a metal, the metal emits electrons. However, up to a certain threshold the metal does not emit electrons, and above this threshold it emits electrons whose energy remains constant. The wave theory of light cannot explain this behaviour.

Einstein suggested that light, previously considered only as an electromagnetic wave, could be described in terms of quanta, or particles that today we call photons. The explanation provided by Einstein treats light in terms of particle beams, rather than in terms of waves, and it opened the way to the wave-particle duality.

Today, the exact equivalent of Young's experiment can be conducted using an electron beam. Electrons launched in a double slit experiment produce an interference pattern on the detector screen and must therefore propagate as waves. However, upon arrival, they generate only one point of light, thus behaving like particles.

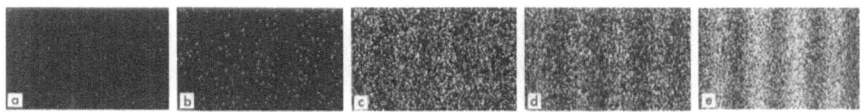

If the electron were a particle it would have to go through one or the other of the two holes in the experiment; however, the interference pattern shows that it behaves as waves that go through the two holes at the same time. According to Richard Feynman in the double-slit experiment, the central mystery of quantum mechanics is hidden:

> *It is a phenomenon in which it is impossible, absolutely impossible, to find a classical explanation, and that well represents the nucleus of quantum*

mechanics. In reality, it contains the only mystery (...) The fundamental peculiarities of all quantum mechanics.

Wave-particle duality is predicted by the theory of syntropy. The theory of syntropy states that there are as many causes as attractors and that nothing happens without the contribution of both. The wave particle duality is a demonstration of the past and future duality, of the duality of causality and retrocausality. The past manifests itself as a particles, while the future as waves. For light to propagate, the past is necessary (the emitter), that is, the particle, but also the future, that is, the wave (the absorber).

Quantum mechanics and special relativity were considered incompatible because they lead to predict the existence of the future that retroacts into the present and the past. In order to explain the wave and particle duality, without resorting to retrocausality and the future, Niels Bohr and Werner Heisenberg proposed the idea that consciousness has the ability to transform the wave into a particle, thus determining the manifestation of reality. According to this interpretation, consciousness precedes and determines reality.

Bohr and Heisenberg were fervent Nazis and their interpretation was used to support the ideology of the Nazi superman. When Schrödinger realized the way in which his wave function had been reinterpreted into a wave of probabilities with mystical connotations, he commented: *"I do not like it, and I never wanted to have anything to do with it!"* Einstein immediately distanced himself by saying that the recourse to consciousness and probability was the proof of the incompleteness of this interpretation.

Soon the scientific debate degraded into an ideological confrontation and in April 1933, during a trip to the United States, Einstein learned that the new German government had enacted a law that excluded Jews from any public office, including university teaching. A month later, on May 10, 1933, the propaganda minister Joseph Goebbels proclaimed that Jewish science was dead and ordered the burning of books, including the works of Einstein.

Einstein's name was on the list of the enemies of the regime that had to be eliminated, and a reward was offered to those who had brought his head. In the German newspapers Einstein was listed among the enemies of the new German regime with the phrase: *"not yet hanged"*. Einstein's publications and books were burned, his villa on the outskirts of Berlin was sacked, his bank account blocked, and his violin destroyed. Hitler had been convinced of the dangers of Jewish science from the book *100 Authors against Einstein.* The theory of relativity was banned and stigmatized as deliriums of an enemy of the Third Reich, conspiracy of Jewish science, while the interpretation of Bohr and Heisenberg became an integral part of the Nazi ideology.

Causality and retrocausality coexist in the quantum world. The retrocausal properties of homeopathy emerge from the quantum world, and use the hydrogen bond of water which bridges the quantum world with the world of materiality in which we live.

The way in which retrocausality operates is reversed with respect to causality. With causality in order to increase the effect, the force of the cause must be increased, as energy dissipates and the effect tends to decrease. With retrocausality to increase the effect, the perturbation must be as small as possible and must be placed near the attractor. It is the attractor that amplifies the effect.

We have already seen that the water molecule, thanks to the hydrogen bridge, acts as a bridge between the quantum world and our macrocosm level. It is for this reason that the properties of water are symmetrical with respect to all other liquids, but it is also for this reason that homeopathic remedies must be based on water and that the greater the dilutions, the more the effects of the remedy are amplified. Dilutions and dynamisations pass the information of the remedy from our molecular level to the quantum level, thus bringing it closer to the attractor that will enhance its effect.

The syntropic properties of retrocausality are very evident in the field of homeopathy, but they can find innumerable applications in many other sectors.

An example, which may appear very distant, allows us to understand why homeopathy must work on the similar. It dates back to 2012 when I was with Antonella in San Francisco to attend a conference of SAND, Science and Non-Duality. In the same days, the baseball final was held in San Francisco, and the San Francisco Giants were one of the worst teams in the American history. We were guests of a friend, one of the most famous healers in the United States who used a technique that he had learned from Nicolai Levashov.

Our friend tried to help the Giants by acting on them using this technique based on the three-dimensional visualization of the person he wanted to help and on the use of the vital energy of his hands in order to dissolve the energy blocks. The effects he achieved with the Giants were disappointing, difficult to evaluate. The Giants continued to lose.

At that point I had the idea to explain him that according to the theory of syntropy, the result is enhanced thanks to the butterfly effect, that is thanks to retrocausality. In practice, I told him to record the game, not to see it and at the end of the game, without knowing the result, to start seeing the recording and proceed with his remote healing technique. He had to act in a retrocausal mode on an already completed game.

As soon as he began to use this retrocausal mode, the Giants started to win, obtaining increasingly surprising results and succeeding in achieving what no other team had ever done before in the history of the American baseball.

There is a short video, shot in San Francisco with our healer friend. The link is youtu.be/ubdNpH-zPwo.

Obviously, it could have been just a coincidence, but we then repeated the experiment in completely different circumstances and on other types of situations, even much more complex, always getting surprising results.

What these experiments tell is that when working in a retrocausal mode one can only help and never oppose. For example, you cannot block the rival team, but you can only facilitate the team you want to help.

While allopathic medicine is based on the principle of opposition, contrasting the symptom and the disease, homeopathic medicine follows the principle of similitude and must facilitate, help the disease to do its job.

There are countless studies and experiments concerning retrocausality. An extract of Antonella's thesis *"Retrocausality, experiments and theory"* is available at: www.amazon.it/dp/1520284225

Homeopathic medicine acts on the invisible plane, the spiritual plane of existence. It is possible to act on this plane also in other ways.

In fact, the fundamental equations show that energy, which is a unity and cannot be neither created nor destroyed (first law of Thermodynamics), is made of an equal amount of syntropic energy and entropic energy. This is written as follows:

$$1 = entropy + syntropy$$

Moving syntropy to the left we have: *syntropy=1-entropy*. In other words, syntropy and entropy are one the complement of the other, they are equal parts of an indivisible unity. This concept is expressed in a masterly way by the figure of the yin and the yang.

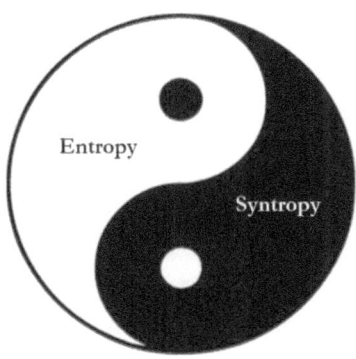

Where entropy and syntropy are part of the same unity and are perfectly balanced. Moreover, within one, we find the other. This leads to describe the universe as a dynamic reality, a continuous dance between entropy and syntropy. Entropy and syntropy are constantly playing together like Shiva and Shakti.

The principle of complementarity between entropy and syntropy can also be represented using a seesaw.

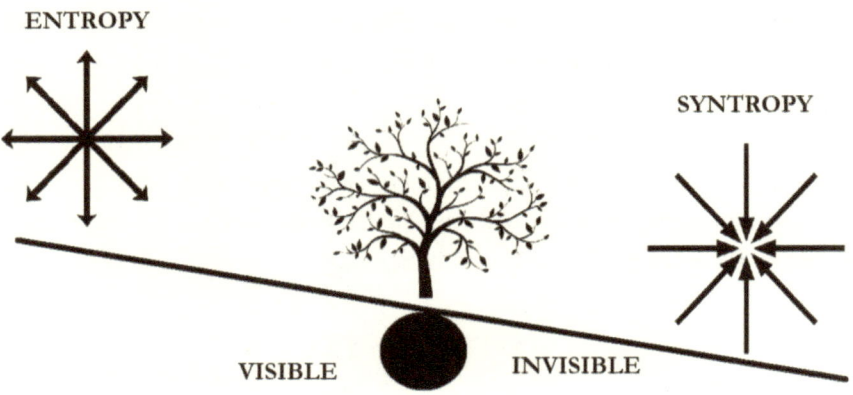

Life is an expression on the physical plane of syntropy and in order to survive, syntropy must increase. However, this is hampered by our activities which, on the contrary, increase entropy. The game of life is just this: how to increase syntropy and reduce entropy by remaining active?

Syntropy activates the processes of the invisible world that enhance life, well-being and wealth. Often, this is thwarted by the fact that people, in order to give meaning to their existence, fall back into entropic lifestyles. This is a problem that is constantly observed and can only be solved by adding an inner work of transformation that allows to respond to the need for meaning no longer by looking outside (through the judgment of others, possession, wealth, power and ideologies), but looking inside (in the heart, through the theorem of love).

To better understand this mechanism, I want to use one of the first cases in which we used this approach. It is about a freelance, single, whose expenses exceeded the income of more than five hundred euro a month! The savings were about to end and he had no one to ask for help. He began to reduce expenses: no money in the wallet, no credit in the mobile phone. But things went from bad to worse. At this point he asked us for help. Let's see how it went.

> «*How much do you spend for your mobile phone?*»
> «*About 40 euros a month, but I always find myself without credit.*»
> «*Why don't you change provider? There are interesting promotions. With only 10 euros a month you can have unlimited minutes and SMS and 20 gigabytes of internet.*»

Lowering entropy is synonymous to saving, but this must be done by maintaining or increasing the quality of life. For example, by modifying an old contract. In this case, changing the telephone company and choosing a contract of the latest generation has led to increase the quality of life and save over three hundred euros a year! The trick is to improve the quality of life by saving money. When entropy and syntropy are balanced the invisible world of syntropy manages to manifest. In this example we have to reduce the spending by at least six thousand euros a year.

> «*Do you take shirts to the laundry to be ironed?*»
> «*I wash them, but I am not able to iron them. I take them to the laundry to have them ironed.*»
> «*How much does it cost you?*»
> «*Between 50 and 70 euros a month.*»
> «*Why don't you ask your maid if she can iron your shirts for an extra 8 euros a month?*»

The maid immediately accepted. Another small optimization that saves more than six hundred euros a year, but which significantly increases the quality of life. In fact, there is no more the hassle of going to the laundry to bring and get the shirts. Again an increase in the quality of life by saving! These first two optimizations have lowered entropy by about a thousand euros a year. We have to get to six thousand euros to balance incomes and outputs, before the magic of the invisible world begins to manifest!

«Do you go to work by car?»
«I also use the scooter, to save money, but the traffic is really dangerous!»
«Why don't you use the bicycle?»
«On these roads?!»
«No, on alternative routes.»
«My house is located in the town centre, the office is not far, but I have always considered the bicycle impossible for the difference in altitude of more than 30 meters. I would arrive tired and sweaty.»
«If you have to climb it's better to choose a steep but short road, get off and push, rather than pedalling.»

He was fascinated by the beauty of the roads of the town centre and the parks. He discovered that in less than 25 minutes he could get to his office by bicycle. Using the car or the scooter it took more time. The day after he sold the scooter, cancelled the insurance and the rent of the garage. In total, another three thousand euros a year saved. With this simple optimization, he received other benefits: he exercises and no longer needs to go to the gym, more money and time saved! Also, he spends less on fuels. Entropy has now decreased by more than four thousand euros a year and the quality of life has improved! We need to find another two thousand euros before syntropy and the invisible world can begin to show.

«Your electricity bill exceeds 200 euros every two months! As a single you

should not pay more than 50 euros.»
«What should I do?»
«Try using low-consumption light bulbs, such as LED lamps, and put the timer to the water heater.»

Small changes that took little time and money. One hundred and fifty euros saved every two months, nine hundred euros a year. With this little optimization he felt happy because of his ecological beliefs and the quality of life increased. Saving energy made him feel consistent with his ideals. Now he has reduced spending of over five thousand euros a year! We need to reach the goal of six thousand euros a year!

«How much do you pay for electricity at your office?»
«About 300 euros every two months.»
«Do you use halogen bulbs!?»
«Yes.»

He discovered that he could save another thousand euros a year by simply replacing the halogen spotlights with LED spotlights. Increasing syntropy means to optimize while increasing the quality of life. Now, spending does no longer exceed incomes. Syntropy can begin to show in the form of synchronicities, which are meaningful coincidences. Jung and Pauli have coined the term synchronicity to indicate an invisible causality different from that familiar to us. Synchronicities manifest as meaningful coincidences, since they converge towards an end.

Invisible causality acts from the future and groups events according to purposes. Synchronicities are meaningful coincidences as they have a purpose.

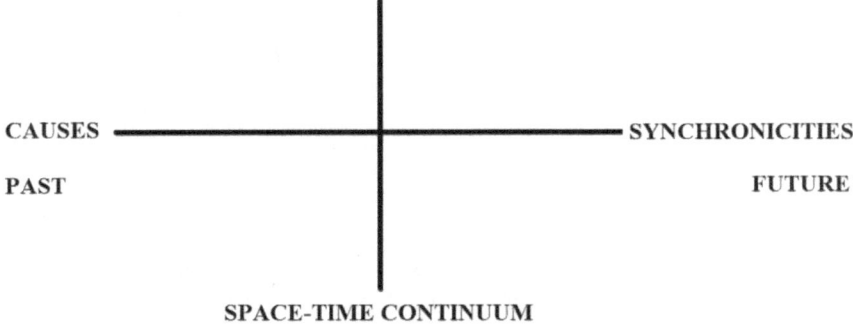

«How much do you pay for renting your office?»
«Nothing. It's owned by my aunts.»
«They could rent it and make a profit, but you use it for free?»
«Exactly.»
«And your aunts on what do they live on?»
«Both have a pension and some savings, but their financial situation is not good, they complain continuously.»
«Have you ever thought about renting a room in an office and letting your aunts rent their apartment?»
«I have no money, I cannot afford to pay a rent!»
«How is your business going?»
«I have few clients, perhaps because of the economic crisis, but also because of the position of the office.»
«A less prestigious office, but in a strategic, well-connected place could help you have more clients?»

The first synchronicity is the following one. The day after this dialogue, as if by magic, he receives the offer of a room in an office in the most central area of the city, at the price of only 250 euros per month, including all utilities! The apartment of the aunts was in a very beautiful and prestigious place, but difficult to reach and there was no parking: beautiful, prestigious, but uncomfortable and very expensive. However he hesitated, he did not dare!

The next day, however, another synchronicity occurred. He

received a call from the doorkeeper. An airline company offered 2,800 euros a month for the apartment of his aunts. The aunts obviously asked him to find another place immediately. Fortunately, the day before he had received the offer of a room. But he was not yet convinced. The office in the centre of town was in a very noisy area: well connected, but chaotic.

The third synchronicity is as follows. That same afternoon he was walking in the area of the city he likes most, not central, but green, quiet and well connected. At the window of a shoemaker, he saw an advertisement for a room for rent in a professional studio. The apartment was in the building next to the shoemaker. He called and immediately went to see it. He instantly decided to rent the room. In a city like Rome it is difficult to find rooms for rent in professional studios and especially in such a beautiful place of the city. When the synchronicities are activated we are attracted to places and situations that otherwise we would not have taken into account and which solve our problems. Synchronicities are accompanied by feelings of warmth and wellbeing in the thoracic area which inform us that we are on the right path.

> «*I began to feel warmth and wellbeing in the thoracic area. My clients liked the new studio. There is parking, the place is nice, quiet and is located near a subway station. My business begun to flourish, my savings have increased and my personal and sentimental life has improved.*»

Syntropy provides wellbeing, happiness and wealth. But when things go well it's easy to fall back into old entropic and dissipative life styles. A few months later, he received an offer of a prestigious work abroad: his dream! He immediately accepted and moved. The salary was high, taxation low. Suddenly he would become a rich man who could lead the rich life he had always dreamed of.

But this reverses the balance of the seesaw: wealth leads to live in an entropic way, entropy increases and syntropy decreases and again we go towards failure and discomfort!

«The foreign company was only interested in making money, no ethics. I had to work almost fifty hours a week, there was nothing else outside the company. One had to give absolute priority to what was profitable, even if immoral. A few months later I felt disgusted of my profession. Taxes were low, but the services were all private. Adding to this the rent of the house and expenses related to the fact that I was a foreigner, I paid much more than I earned. After only six months I had accumulated more than twenty-eight thousand euros in debts. The dream had shattered and had become a nightmare. From heaven I had fallen to hell. I had no time for myself or my emotional and relational life. I first felt discomfort, then suffering, and finally depression and anguish exploded. I decided to come back to Italy!»

It often happens this way. Increasing syntropy increases the quality of life, wellbeing and wealth. But, as soon as material wealth returns, the person falls into an entropic life style and returns again into misery.

The increase in syntropy must be accompanied by an inner change. People must not consider money as their property, but as a tool. They must be aware that happiness and realization are not achieved through materiality, but thanks to love, to the Theorem of Love.

If this change is lacking, the process fails. Material improvements must be accompanied by inner changes towards syntropy. Wealth is just one aspect of the game between entropy and syntropy. When wealth is obtained without an inner transformation it is inevitable to fall back into entropy and suffering.

This game between entropy and syntropy is played not only by individuals, but also by societies and nations. It can be successfully used in the management of a city, a nation, public and private organizations, in ecological and natural systems. But it must always be accompanied by an inner transformation, otherwise it eventually leads to failure, to an increase in entropy.

3

INTUITIONS

Syntropy is energy that converges. The system that is responsible for the acquisition of syntropy is the neurovegetative system and for this reason we feel syntropy as a sensation of warmth and well-being in the thoracic area.

When we converge towards the attractor and the acquisition of syntropy is good, we perceive warmth and well-being in the thoracic area due to a good inflow of syntropy and a good support of the vital processes. On the contrary when we diverge from the attractor the acquisition of syntropy is insufficient and we perceive void, pain and feelings of death due to a poor support of the vital life functions.

The feelings of warmth in the thorax area are commonly referred to as love and happiness, while those of void and pain as distress, angst and anxiety.

These feelings offer important information about the attractor as they behave like a compass. When we are converging towards the attractor, we feel warmth and well-being, while when we diverge we feel anguish and pain.

In this regard, the neurologist Antonio Damasio, who has studied people affected by decision-making deficit, has discovered that these feelings contribute to the decision-making process and make it possible to make advantageous choices without having to make advantageous assessments. It seems that cognitive processes have been added to emotional ones, maintaining the centrality of emotions in decision-making. This is evident in the moments of danger: when choices must be made quickly, reason is bypassed.

Patients affected by decision-making deficits are characterized by knowledge but not by feeling. Their cognitive functions are intact, but not the emotional ones. These patients are endowed with normal intellect, but they are not able to decide appropriately. There is a dissociation between rational skills and decision-making skills. The alteration of inner feelings causes a form of short-sightedness towards the future. It can be caused by neurological injuries or the use of substances, such as alcohol and heroin, that alter the perception of inner feelings.

The importance of these inner feelings was described by Henri Poincaré, one of the most creative mathematicians of the last century. Poincaré noted that when faced with a new problem whose solutions are potentially infinite, he initially used the rational approach, but then not being able to arrive to the solution, another type of process became necessary. This process selected the correct solution among all the infinite possibilities, without the help of rationality. Poincaré named it intuition (from the Latin words *in*=inner + *tueri*=look), and was struck by the fact that intuitions were always accompanied by a feeling of truth, beauty, warmth and well-being in the thoracic area:

Among the large number of possible combinations,
almost all are without interest or utility.
Only those that lead to solving the problem are noticed by the conscience
because they are accompanied by an inner experience of truth and beauty.

For Poincaré the process of intuition is amplified when we learn to pay attention to these inner feelings.

According to syntropy these inner feelings connect us to the attractor and play a very important role allowing us to identify solutions and the purpose of our existence.

Steve Jobs, the founder of Apple Computer, provided an important example.

Steve Jobs was always trying to reduce entropy in an obsessive way. After he got married it took him more than 8 months to choose the washing machine. He absolutely had to find the one with the lowest entropy, which consumed the less. He lived in a frugal and minimalist way. A life so essential and Spartan to bring his children to believe that he was a poor man. The way he lived was the result of choices that led him to focus on the heart, on the inner feelings. He avoided wealth, because it could distract him from the inner feelings, the inner voice of the heart. He became one of the richest men on the planet, but he lived like a poor man! His minimalist choices were necessary to enhance his intuitions, the source of his wealth.

Steve Jobs had been abandoned by his natural parents and this was a drama that accompanied him throughout his whole life. He was tormented, he never accepted that he had been abandoned. He quit university during the first semester of the first year and ventured to India to look for himself. He returned with a totally changed vision of the world. The trip to India marked the change. He discovered that in the Indian countryside people do not let themselves be guided by rationality, as we do, but by intuitions, by focusing on the heart. He described intuitions as a very powerful faculty, very developed in India, but practically unknown in the West.

He returned to the States convinced that intuitions are more powerful than the intellect. In order to cultivate intuitions it was necessary an essential life, a vegan diet, free of animal products, abstention from alcohol, tobacco and coffee, meditation and the courage not to be influenced by the judgment of others

Jobs opposed marketing studies, as he believed that people do not know their future. Only intuitive people can feel the future. When he returned to the United States he saw an electronic board at Steve Wozniak's home and he had the intuition of a computer that could be held in one hand, a smartphone. Going against the opinion of everyone, he asked Wozniak to develop a prototype of a personal computer, which he named Apple I. He managed to sell a few hundred of them and this sudden success gave Steve Jobs the push to develop a more advanced model, suitable for ordinary people, which he called Apple II.

Jobs was not an engineer, he did not have a scientific or technical mind, he was simply an artist! What did computers have to do with his life? Jobs had nothing to do with computers and electronics, but his intuitive abilities showed him an object of the future. Thirty years in advance, back in 1977, he had the intuition of the smartphone: a pocket computer that combines aesthetics with technology and minimalism! He sensed the need for a product that in addition to being technologically perfect was also beautiful and simple!

His obsession with beauty and simplicity led him to spend a lot of time designing the case of Apple II. It had to be beautiful, silent and at the same time essential and simple! It was an unprecedented business success that made Apple one of the leading companies on a global scale.

Jobs says that when the heart gave him an insight for him this became a diktat. It had to be done, regardless of the opinions of others. The only thing that mattered was finding a way to give shape to the intuition.

For Jobs, the vegan diet, Zen meditation, a life immersed in nature, abstaining from alcohol and coffee were necessary choices in order to have a pure heart, to nourish his inner voice, the voice of his heart and strengthen in this way the intuitive abilities. At the same time, this caused great difficulties. He was sensitive, intuitive, but irrational. He was aware of the limits that his irrationality gave him in managing a large company, like Apple Computer. He therefore put rationalist managers at the direction of his company, such as John Sculley, a famous manager whom he himself admired, but with whom he continually came into conflict. To the point that in 1985 the board of directors decided to fire Jobs from Apple Computer, the company that he had founded.

The company continued for a while to make money on the products that Jobs had designed, but after a few years the decline began. In the mid-nineties, Apple Computer was in crisis and had come to the brink of bankruptcy. On December 21, 1996, the board of directors asked Jobs to return as a personal adviser to the president. Jobs accepted. He demanded a salary of one dollar a year in exchange for the guarantee that his insights, though crazy, were accepted unconditionally. In a few months he revolutionized the products and on September 16, 1997 he became CEO ad interim. Apple Computer resurrected in less than a year.

How did he manage?

He repeated that we must not allow the noise of other people's opinions cloud our inner voice. And more importantly, he repeated that we must always have the courage to believe in our heart and intuitions, as they already know the future and know where we have to go. For Jobs everything else was secondary. His being at interim marked all his new products. He wanted their name to be preceded by the letter *i*: *i*Pod, *i*Pad, *i*Phone and *i*Mac.

Jobs led a minimalist life. His children believed that he was a poor man. Often his children asked: *"Daddy, why don't you take us to one of your rich friends?"* He talked about important business walking in the parks or in the middle of nature. To celebrate success, he invited in restaurants for 10 dollars per person. He did not drink alcohol and when he had to make a present he collected flowers in a field. He wore the same clothes for years. Despite the immense fortunes he had!

He believed that money was not his, but that it served to reach an end. At the time of Apple I, he repeated that his mission was to develop a computer that could be held in one hand and not to become rich. For him money was exclusively a tool. The ability to feel was the source of Jobs's wealth. It was the ingredient of his creativity, genius and innovation. Einstein used to say that the intuitive mind is a sacred gift and the rational mind is its faithful servant. But we have created a society that honours the servant and has forgotten the gift.

Zen meditation helped Jobs to calm the chatter of the mind and shift attention to the heart.

In his lectures, Jobs used to say that almost everything: expectations, pride and fears of bankruptcy, vanish in front of death. He constantly emphasized the centrality of death and the fact that death leaves only what is really important. Remembering that we must die was the best way for him to understand what was really important and to avoid the trap of sticking to materiality. Remembering that we are already naked before death gives the strength not to be afraid. Since we have to die there is no reason not to follow the heart.

Jobs believed very much in the invisible and in synchronicities. For this reason he built the headquarters of Apple around a central space, a large piazza where everyone had to go through or stop if they wanted to consume something or use the services. In this way the invisible world of intuitions and creativity was favoured by chance encounters. According to Jobs, chance does not exist and in a piazza chance meetings allow the invisible, synchronicities, to activate intuitions and the creativity abilities of the invisible world. Intuitions and aesthetic sensibility make visible what is not yet visible.

Jobs loved Michelangelo's famous sentence:

In every block of marble I see a statue as plain as though it stood before me, shaped and perfect in attitude and action. I have only to hew away the rough walls that imprison the lovely apparition to reveal it to the other eyes as mine see it.

Jobs believed that everyone has a task, a mission to carry out. We just have to rediscover this mission removing all that is not necessary. Jobs made visible what he had sensed. He died a few months after presenting the *i*Phone, the computer held in one hand, the mission of his life.

His life testifies that intelligence and creativity come from the invisible world and that we can access the invisible world through intuitions. He showed that the voice of the heart makes it possible to feel the future.

All that operates on the invisible side, and therefore also homeopathy, must give great attention to intuitions. Finding the right remedy is not a mechanical task, but it is the result of processes that are also intuitive and that no one will ever be able to code in a manual.

4

EPILOGUE

The invisible world of life energy works in a reversed way compared to the ordinary visible material reality: in order to become rich we must live frugally, to unite we must maximize diversity, to be incisive we must reduce the force. This allows to accomplish tasks that would otherwise be impossible.

A question is often asked: *Do attractors, ends, mean that the future is already determined?*

No. Attractors are the point from which syntropy emanates, the vital and cohesive energy, and to which we must converge. However, the route depends on our choices. If there were no attractors we would only be the product of the past: totally determined machines. We are free. Our life is not determined, because we must continually choose whether to follow the head or the heart, the past or the future.

The error lies in considering the past certain and fixed and the future as non-existent. We limit ourselves to the causes, to linear rational thinking that increase entropy, suffering, crises and illnesses.

Healing requires a change of paradigm, a shift from a mechanistic view, of cause and effect, to a new supercausal vision in which we must continually mediate between causes and attractors, in which the future retroacts on the present and can be felt thanks to intuitions and insights.

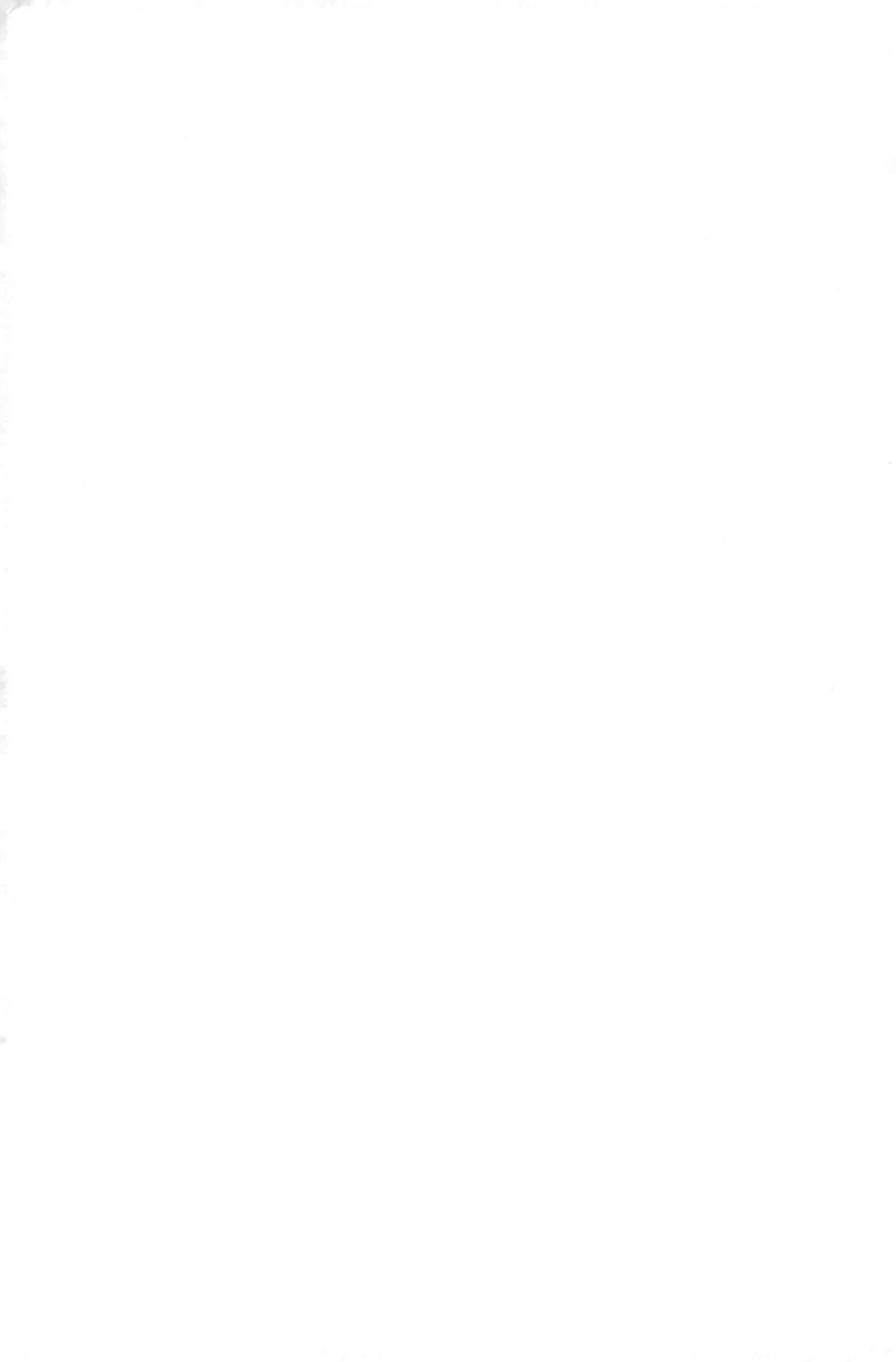

www.ingramcontent.com/pod-product-compliance
Lightning Source LLC
Chambersburg PA
CBHW030452220526
45464CB00006B/2504